Acceptable Prejudice?

Fat, Rhetoric
and
Social Justice

Lonie McMichael, Ph.D.

PEARLSONG PRESS
NASHVILLE, TN

PEARLSONG PRESS | P.O. BOX 58065 | NASHVILLE, TN 37205
www.pearlsong.com | www.pearlsongpress.com

Trade paperback ISBN: 9781597190657 | Ebook ISBN: 9781597190640

Book & cover design by Zelda Pudding

The essay "How to Support Fat Acceptance as a Thin Person" is a condensed version of posts originally published on the blog *Unapologetically Fat* and is © 2013 Jo Conklin, a.k.a. Jo Geek. Spelling, punctuation and word usage in blog posts and quotations and the preferred noncapitalization of some names have been preserved in this book, with the exception of the occasional correction of apparent typos and capitalization of names at the start of sentences or in chapter or section titles. Health At Every Size® and HAES℠ are registered trademarks and service marks of the Association for Size Diversity and Health and are used with permission.

ALSO BY LONIE MCMICHAEL
Talking Fat: Health vs. Persuasion in the War on Our Bodies

Book group study guides to *Acceptable Prejudice?* and *Talking Fat* can be downloaded from www.pearlsong.com/acceptableprejudice.htm and www.pearlsong.com/talkingfat.htm.

Library of Congress Cataloging-in-Publication Data

McMichael, Lonie, 1966–
   Acceptable prejudice? : fat, rhetoric and social justice / Lonie McMichael, Ph.D.
        pages cm
   Includes bibliographical references.
   ISBN 978-1-59719-065-7 (trade pbk. : alk. paper)—ISBN 978-1-59719-064-0 (ebook)
   1. Discrimination against overweight persons. 2. Physical-appearance-based bias. 3. Obesity—Social aspects. I. Title.
   RC628.M379 2013
   362.1963'98—dc23
                                                    2013010508

To all the fat activists
For your courage—
For your willingness—
For your heart—
You folks are my heroes

Contents

Acknowledgements

Like my previous book, *Talking Fat: Health vs. Persuasion in the War on Our Bodies,* I would never have finished this work without the aid of two people who are very special to me: my dissertation chair, Amy Koerber, and my partner, Tully Dozier. Thank you both for your support and your confidence in me!

Also, I would like to thank Erec Smith, a colleague in fat studies and rhetoric who took his own precious time to review this book and help me out with intersectionality issues.

Introduction

Fat prejudice has doubled in the last decade within the U.S., yet even progressives refuse to believe fat individuals deserve protection from oppression. Fat individuals walk through life at times being told that they are unlovable and unworthy, being denied jobs and experiences, and being shunned by society, all the while being told they are at fault—if they want it to change, just lose weight. However, we have no scientific evidence that it is possible to lose weight permanently. We do have a great deal of evidence that fat is a normal part of human diversity.

I am writing this book for a few reasons. First off, I want fat individuals in America to understand that yes, you do experience prejudice and domination—prejudice and domination that is not justified. To that end I attempt to document the experiences of several fat individuals. Fat individuals tend to buy into the belief that they deserve poor treatment, a process called internalization. I want fat individuals to understand how that internalization happens and how to overcome it. Using the experiences of fat individuals who have overcome the negative beliefs about themselves, I provide a guide for making peace with the fat body.

I am also writing this book to hold feminist and social justice advocates who believe fat individuals do not deserve protection responsible for buying into the belief of the kierarchy—the hierarchy of dominance including patriarchy, white supremacy, etc.—that fat is bad. Fat prejudice is alive and well and being practiced on a daily basis by those who eschew all other forms of prejudice.

One myth heard about fat is that it is the last acceptable prejudice. For instance, Rebecca Puhl and Kelly Brownell, researchers of fat stigma at the Rudd Center for Food Policy and Obesity, say in their book *Weight Bias* that fat is the "last acceptable basis of discrimination." Ask any transgendered individual and they will tell you otherwise. Racism and sexism may be overtly rejected in our society, but covertly they are still prevalent. Ask any individual who is physically disabled and they will tell you of their experiences in terms of oppression and prejudice, since they face prejudice and stigma on a daily basis. Folks with mental health issues face stigma all the time. Other prejudices and stigmas exist, and we are creating new ones regularly. People who look different, by choice or not, are often the subject of preconceived negative attitudes—they are defined as "Other," as somehow not human. It is apparent that fat is NOT the last acceptable prejudice; acceptable prejudices abound.

The reason fat is called the last acceptable prejudice is that even many social justice advocates believe that fat individuals deserve the stigma they face. Where a joke about a little person or a racial slur will get you chastised by a social justice advocate, fat prejudice and oppression are seldom questioned. This book is an attempt to bring awareness to liberals and feminists; far too many people who put themselves in the social justice category believe that fat individuals deserve the treatment they receive.

Finally, I want to clarify how prejudice works, building on the ideas of Gloria Jean Watkins, who writes as bell hooks (she intentionally does not capitalize her pen name). One day as a society we will understand that fat prejudice, along with all other stigmas, is not acceptable. However, if we do not understand how domination works we will find our society justifying yet another prejudice—and that is unacceptable. It is time for Western society to understand that no prejudice is EVER acceptable. It is time for us to see all people as individuals and none as inhuman "Other." It is time for us to grow up and become a mature, accepting society.

My hope is that through the reading of this book the reader will question how our society treats those who do not fit the "norm," those who stand out as different. Prejudice, stigma and oppression are not acceptable in enlightened societies, as the United States claims to be. It is time for us to recognize all oppression, even well-hidden oppression, and put a stop to it. It is time for us to become a truly enlightened society.

FOUNDATIONAL CONCEPTS

In this book I will use some terms and names that you may not be familiar with or that may be used in ways you have not heard before. To start, I will explain these terms and how I use them within my work.

CHAPTER 1
Hooks' Ideology of Domination

To understand fat prejudice I used bell hooks' ideology of domination (so termed by rhetors Sonja K. Foss, Karen A. Foss and Robert Trapp) as a lens, examining the experience of fat individuals in Western culture through hooks' concepts around prejudice and oppression. Hooks proposed this philosophy to explain a social dynamic of prejudice and domination within American society—specifically, that our culture includes those who are considered privileged and acceptable while other people are considered substandard or second-rate, with the privileged dominating the others.

Hooks calls the dominating forces "the white supremacist patriarchy." In this book I use the term "kierarchy" instead. The term "kierarchy" (also spelled "kyriarchy") was coined by progressive theologian Elisabeth Schussler Fiorenza to describe the dominating forces viewed as "the elite" in American society. Examples of "the elite" forces include patriarchy, racial oppression, and socio-economic oppression. I use the term "kierarchy" to emphasize the expanse of domination in our society.

In hooks' ideology she contends that the oppressed, the dominated, "internalize and enforce the values" of the dominant regime, helping to perpetuate the prevailing dynamic. She notes that the dominated "can and do participate in politics of domination, as perpetrators as well as victims—that we dominate, that we are dominated." Though hooks believes this is primarily a Western phenomenon, she asserts that our society, possibly even the world, is governed by this ideology of domination:

> We live in a world in crisis—a world governed by politics of domination, one in which the belief in a notion of superior and inferior, and its concomitant ideology—that the superior should rule over the inferior—affects the lives of all people everywhere...

As a solution to this dynamic of domination hooks offers what she calls "love." Her concept of love is not the sentimental feeling we usually associate with the term, but rather a force that fights against dehumanization, according to Foss, Foss and Trapp.

She claims that "to be either dominated or dominating is a point of connection, of commonality," providing a common ground for ending domination. Such dynamics of domination should be completely eradicated, in hooks' view:

> Therefore, it is necessarily a struggle to eradicate the ideology of domination that permeates Western culture on various levels, as well as a commitment to reorganizing society so that the self-development of people can take precedence over imperialism, economic expansion, and material desires.

"Colonization" is a word hooks often uses to explain this idea of domination. When oppressed individuals come to believe that they are bad for having the qualities that make them oppressed, their minds become colonized, hooks argues. She believes that to resist the internal messages of inferiority, oppressed individuals must decolonize, or free, their minds.

I contend that we can find this same dynamic, this ideology

of domination, being played out currently in the American society around fat. Throughout this book I apply hooks' concepts to the fat experience, looking specifically at how this ideology functions in the lives of fat individuals. I show that fat individuals internalize the belief in their own inferiority, learn to resist that internal belief, learn to resist external messages of inferiority, and finally find that love is the solution to prejudice and domination.

Any and all forms of domination are a problem and should be eradicated, hooks believes. She calls the interrelation of capitalism and race, class and gender oppression the "politic of domination:"

> [T]he ideological ground that they share, which is a belief in domination, and a belief in the notions of superior and inferior, which are components of all of those systems. For me it's like a house, they share the foundation, but the foundation is the ideological beliefs around which notions of domination are constructed.

To overcome this domination those in the margin, those being oppressed, must be "understood, addressed, and incorporated." She encourages the elimination of such domination everywhere and in all ways.

I use bell hooks' concepts and ideas on prejudice and domination to examine the experience of fat individuals. Fat people are experiencing domination to a great degree, yet many individuals in the social justice community are ignoring that fact. Thus I decided to delve into fat using hooks' ideology as a lens for examining the fat experience within American society.

CHAPTER 2
Rhetoric & Fat

I specialize in rhetoric. This concept is important when dealing with society's attitudes on fat, since rhetoric—both visual and verbal—provides the essential medium through which people become prejudiced toward fat people. Rhetoric is also the medium by which people resist that prejudice.

The processes by which a fat individual internalizes negative views of fat and in turn resists negative views of fat are rooted in rhetoric. I contend that prejudice originates in the words and images fat individuals confront from childhood on. But because prejudice is rhetorical, we can use rhetoric to fight its effects.

What is rhetoric? Rhetorician Jack Selzer believes that no common definition of rhetoric exists. However, in the Western tradition, Aristotle's definition of rhetoric as "the faculty of observing in any given case the available means of persuasion" is often treated as the authority. Rhetorical scholars tend to associate rhetoric "with the means of producing effective discursive acts"—in other words, rhetoric comes from communication and discussion.

Using a conglomeration of these ideas, I interpret rhetoric as persuasive acts of communication. As I show throughout this book, fat prejudice is rooted in such communication, as is resistance to fat prejudice.

Science Rhetoric & Fat

The rhetoric of fat pervades our society, as evidenced by the popularity of the topic of "obesity" in the dominant culture of the United States today. This rhetoric comes from scientific texts based in empirical research conducted by experts and published in peer-reviewed journals. But it also comes from pseudo-scientific texts that have no empirical backing, yet bear the ethos of science because they are associated with or penned by an individual who is seen as an expert.

Medical studies are often simplified and presented to the general population through the media—print and online newspapers, news sites, and magazines—which changes the message to be "more human-oriented and better suited for increasing the narrative potential or emotionality of scientific news than for raising or adjudicating questions about its validity," says journalist and professor Susan MacDonald.

To understand the rhetoric of fat I look at the messages fat individuals receive from family, friends, health-care providers, society as a whole, and even strangers. By understanding these messages I seek to understand how fat prejudice works.

In this book I also examine the way fat individuals resist such rhetoric and solutions for fat prejudice itself. To understand how such prejudice functions, I used hooks' ideology of domination to situate my research and reflections.

Hooks' Ideology of Domination & Rhetoric

For hooks' ideology to be relevant in this work we must understand how this ideology is rhetorical. In other words, we need to understand the role of communication in the domination dynamic. As hooks argues, language plays an important part in both the process of internalization and in resisting the dominant rhetoric:

> We are rooted in language, wedded, have our being in words. Language is also a place of struggle. The oppressed struggle in language to recover ourselves—to rewrite, to reconcile, to renew. Our words are not without meaning. They are an action—a resistance. Language is also a place of struggle.

> Dare I speak to oppressed and oppressor in the same voice? Dare I speak to you in a language that will take us away from the boundaries of domination, a language that will not fence you in, bind you, or hold you. Language is also a place of struggle. The oppressed struggle in language to read ourselves—to reunite, to reconcile, to renew. Our words are not without meaning. They are an action—a resistance. Language is also a place of struggle.

Persuasive language and other forms of rhetoric reinforce the dominant values, according to hooks. This situation leads the oppressed individual to internalize, or to assimilate, the belief in their own inferiority. However, language, especially persuasive language, can also be a source of resisting these messages of inferiority. Hooks' ideology of domination is embedded in ideas surrounding discourse and language, especially in relation to persuasion. Understanding the part that language plays in domination and resistance makes it a rhetorical idea.

CHAPTER 3
Fat, Fat Acceptance, Fat Pride & Fat Liberation

"Fat" is a dirty word in our society. We use euphemisms like "large," "big," "curvy," "zaftig," "fluffy" (fluffy—really?), and "thick" to avoid that nasty, nasty word. The word has become an insult and an attack. So when attempting to name their entity, fat activists chose to call their fight "fat acceptance," reclaiming the word "fat" simply as a descriptor like "tall" or "brown-haired." As a shortcut they often refer to the movement as FA. (For more information on the controversy around the name "fat acceptance," see Chapter 13: The Power of Rhetoric).

So what exactly is the fat acceptance movement? No official fat acceptance community exists, though unorganized fat acceptance communities exist both in real life and on the Web.

For the most part, fat acceptance is a grassroots movement that has grown out of feminism in the United States, according to scholars and editors Esther Rothblum and Sondra Solovay in *The Fat Studies Reader*. Individuals within this movement are fighting for the acceptance of size diversity, the acceptance of people of every size—thin, fat and everywhere between. Marilyn Wann uses the term the "fat pride community," while others call it the "fat liberation movement," according to Rothblum and Solovay.

Some individuals in the community have started arguing with the term "fat acceptance." To be accepted, they believe, is not enough. Marilyn Wann has been arguing this point for years. Blogger Kath Read, a.k.a. Fat Heffalump, explains why she doesn't like the term "fat acceptance":

> It is my belief that we more than simply exist on this planet. We have value. We contribute. We are as worthy of our place on the planet as any other human being. Fat people are as precious and worthy as any other human being. We are not damaged goods that need repair. Nor are we "too big" and need to be made smaller to "fit in." The world is big enough for all of us, from the very largest person down to the tiniest. We are not vermin to be eradicated, diseases to be cured or crimes to be prevented. We are people who hold as much value as any other human being on the planet.

> The word "acceptance" makes me feel like I have to compromise my value, because as a fat person I am devalued. And I want no part of that.

I support the concepts of fat pride and fat liberation. However, because many of the participants in my research use the term "fat acceptance," or FA for short, I will use all of the terms above.

Though an organized fat acceptance community does not exist, a few organizations are associated with fat acceptance: the National Association to Advance Fat Acceptance (NAAFA), NOLOSE, and the Association for Size Diversity and Health (ASDAH). NAAFA's website says it is a "civil rights organization dedicated to ending size discrimination in all of its forms" and was founded in 1969 as an outgrowth of the feminist movement during that time. NOLOSE "started out as the *National Organization for Lesbians of SizE* before expanding scope to a broader community of all genders, bound by a common queer, feminist, and fat-positive ideology," according to its website, and is "a vibrant community of fat queers and our allies, with a shared commitment to feminist, anti-oppression ideology and action, seeking to end the oppression of fat people." ASDAH is an association of health information and health care specialists who focus on the idea of Health At Every Size (HAES), a health intervention approach with a more successful track record than dieting (see Chapter 17: Love in Action: Health At Every Size for more information on the HAES philosophy).

After existing for a long time, as NAAFA's foundation date attests, fat acceptance communities have experienced resurgence with the current societal push against fat as well as the advent of the web. Fat positive communities on the web are called the Fatosphere, a very loose conglomeration of blog spaces, discussion boards, Facebook pages, Tumblr pages, Twitter users, etc. who connect online to discuss and support each other on fat matters.

The term "Fatosphere" was originally popularized by blogger FatFu, according to Kate Harding, a once very popular blogger on the Fatosphere and co-author of *Lessons from the Fat-o-sphere: Quit Dieting and Declare a Truce with Your Body*. FatFu founded the "Notes from the Fatosphere" RSS feed in 2007. Since then the Fatosphere has had blogs and bloggers come and go, while fat liberation advocates and communities can be found on almost all social networks. In fact, much of the current (2012-13) online activity can be found on Twitter and Tumblr on sites such as *Fat Body Politics* and *This is Thin Privilege*. These communities are diverse and different, though some similarities may be found within them—similarities I will address throughout this book.

CHAPTER 4
Background of the Project

I started exploring fat acceptance in 2003, just as I went back to school for a master's degree in technical communication. During a modern rhetoric course I was introduced to the ideas of bell hooks, specifically her ideology of domination. I could easily see how the fat experience fit into her ideology.

So when I went on to pursue my Ph.D. I decided to write a dissertation on that exact idea: how does fat fit with hooks' ideology of domination? In the process of exploring this idea I studied medical and psychosocial research about fat, rhetorically analyzed blogs in the Fatosphere, and interviewed fat individuals who experienced such domination.

All of this research culminated in a dissertation that earned me a Ph.D. in technical communication and rhetoric, and produced two books: *Talking Fat: Health vs. Persuasion in the War on our Bodies* and this book. During that time bloggers and voices in fat acceptance have come and gone, the powers that be have increased their push against fat, and people have started to question the efficacy of trying to lose weight. However, fat prejudice is still occurring frequently within our society.

In this book I examine fat prejudice using bell hooks' ideology of domination by looking specifically at how the process of prejudice works. I scrutinize the experience of fat individuals in relation to this ideology. I also examine the reasons that fat prejudice is either ignored or is accepted as valid.

Now that I have explained the concepts I will be using throughout this book and how I will be using them, we need to explore the basics of fat prejudice in order to understand how such prejudice works in our society.

THE BASICS
OF FAT PREJUDICE

Fat prejudice is thriving in the dominant culture of the United States.
The dominant messages stating that fat is bad, and consequently allowing fat prejudice to exist, are accepted for the
most part even by progressives. As Paul Campos, law professor
and author of *The Diet Myth,* conveyed on NPR:

> Normally, traditionally, especially among political
> progressives, the reaction to social discrimination has not
> been let's get rid of the people being socially discriminated
> against, and that's how we're going to cure this supposed
> problem.

The majority of people in our society, even those who think
they would never condone prejudice, expect fat individuals
to change in order to overcome oppression. In response, we
must ask the question, "How can we, a supposedly enlightened
society, allow such prejudice to exist with so little opposition?"
We allow this prejudice to exist because of many reasons,
including our ideas of health and our attitudes toward prejudice
overall.

CHAPTER 5
The Myth of Justified Oppression

We allow these prejudices to continue because of two myths: Fat is unhealthy in and of itself, and anyone can be thin permanently if they eat right and exercise.

The kierarchy is incredibly skilled at finding ways to cunningly practice prejudice and oppression. Fat individuals know this well, since the kierarchy has succeeded at justifying prejudice towards fat individuals to the point that even most progressives hold such prejudice.

The Myth of Fat as Changeable

The underlying reason for justifying this prejudice lies in the belief that fat is permanently changeable. We have not, however, found a method that keeps weight off for the majority of individuals. This includes both weight loss diets and lifestyle changes. Even when continuing weight loss behaviors, exercise science professor Wayne C. Miller has found, the majority of participants gain the lost weight back. A meta study (a study of studies) by Traci Mann and others actually shows that most people gain back more weight than they originally lost within three years of ending a diet. Bariatric or "weight loss" surgery has slightly better odds, but also has high levels of complications and deaths. Also, we must remember that in bariatric surgery "success" is considered a 10 percent weight loss, which still leaves most surgery victims in the "obese" category.

Studying the medical rhetoric surrounding "obesity," I have found that our society refuses to see a pretty solid truth: fat is seldom permanently eradicated. Our bodies are made to hold onto weight, not to let weight go. Some people believe there is a magic way to lose weight, and we have just not yet found the right combination of foods and exercises. Evidence suggests otherwise.

In the interim, even progressives see a fat person as faulty rather than society as failing. But stigma and oppression will never go away as long as the responsibility to change is on the oppressed. As Ragen Chastain, professional dancer and author of *Fat: The Owner's Manual,* states, "I think that the cure for stigmatization is to change culture and end stigma, not to insist that members of the stigmatized group change themselves so that they can get the approval of the stigmatizing group."

Oppression for Your Own Good, or the Myth of Fat in Itself as Unhealthy

In the last couple of decades we have experienced a major push to eradicate fat people that is set in the guise of "healthy living. From every angle—work, school, media, etc.—we continually receive the message that fat people must lose weight in order to be healthy. However, unbiased researchers discover that fat is not so bad. In fact, fat can have the following protective qualities:

- Fat protects a patient post-operatively. "Overweight" and "obese" individuals have a decreased risk of death in post-surgical ICU.

- "Obese" patients with Type 2 diabetes have lower mortality rates—meaning they live longer.

- Higher mortality is associated with weight loss in Type 2 diabetic patients, yet weight gain did not change mortality rates.

- "Obese" individuals with Type 2 diabetes have fewer incidences of amputation. They also experience better post-operative outcomes after amputation.

- Being "overweight" or "obese" lowers the mortality rate for those with cardiovascular disease.

- "Obesity" protects against respiratory failure in post-operative patients.

- "Obese" dialysis patients have better survival outcomes.

- Chronic Obstructive Pulmonary Disease (COPD) patients with a higher BMI live longer.

- A number of studies reveal that fat individuals have better outcomes after a stroke.

- Weight gain has been associated with lower mortality rates, while weight loss has been associated with higher mortality rates.

Additionally, studies have found that "obese" individuals live about as long as "normal" weight individuals, and "overweight" individuals live the longest. "Underweight" individuals have the shortest life spans. This result was found in three independent studies that took place in the United States, in Canada, and in Japan.

As we can see by this research, "obesity" on its own—a person just being fat—does not cause health problems.

Yet it is an absolute miracle that more fat people are not terribly unhealthy. We know that dieting causes horrible effects to the body, including gallstones and increases in cortisol level. Moreover, the research of Peter Muennig, a medical researcher out of Columbia University, suggests that it is *fat stigma* rather than fat itself that causes the health problems associated with fat.

All the statistics on fat people being unhealthy are worthless because you cannot separate fat from fat stigma. If fat people have issues with health, which is in question, we cannot prove whether it's the actual body fat or the fat stigma that cause them. The issues might completely disappear if fat stigma is successfully obliterated.

The people who are supposed to be helping fat individuals become healthy are some of the most prejudiced out there. Physicians notoriously see fat patients as noncompliant, or unwilling to follow doctors' directions. Forty percent of doctors have been found to have weight prejudice.

Many of the participants in my research have reported poor treatment at the hands of physicians and other health care professionals. I have received numerous reports of individuals who were told to lose weight to solve a problem, only to find out that they had something else going on. I have also found fat individuals who have had weight loss regimes pushed on them when going to the doctor for something completely different (See Chapter 8: Fat People As Inferior for more information on medical prejudice). Since health care practitioners tend to be fat prejudiced, fat individuals tend to receive poor health care.

Ben Spatz, artistic director of Urban Research Theater, articulately states the following on the blog *Cacophony:* "At this point, none of us can tease the scientific or medical facts apart from the cultural revulsion attached to fatness."

We think our push to eliminate fat is about health, but it really, really isn't. The belief that fat reduction is about health has justified and expanded prejudice and oppression. We must change this paradigm, or fat prejudice will continue to expand. Ragen Chastain makes the following argument:

> [S]ee people talk a lot about how we need to "do something" because so many people are "suffering from obesity." I won't presume to speak for everyone but I will say that while I sometimes do suffer because I'm obese, I've never suffered from obesity.

> I'm suffering from living in a society where I'm shamed, stigmatized and humiliated because of the way I look.

So we are being shamed for our own good. For example, many people believe that shaming fat children is an effective way to make them skinny, as exemplified by the Strong4Life campaign out of Georgia. Fat people often experience "drive-by insults" or worse when they are attempting to exercise. In my research I have found reports of fat people out for a walk who had trash or milk shakes thrown at them. This isn't shaming for our own good—this is bullying and prejudice. As a blog commenter named Diann Arcana Johns states in a response to a post about making fun of fat people, "We need to stay in our houses until we're thin, then we can come out and be patted on the back and learn the secret handshake."

So we don't know how to make anyone thin, and fat reduction isn't really about health. What we do know, as unbiased scholars are finding, is that there is a clear correlation between healthy behaviors and healthy bodies no matter the body size. See the next section on the HAES philosophy for more information on how healthy behaviors make healthy bodies, no matter the body size.

For more information on health and fat, see my first book, *Talking Fat: Health vs. Persuasion in the War on our Bodies*.

Health at Every Size (HAES)

The HAES approach is a way to look at health that does not include weight.

Our society's focus on weight as an indicator of health has two major implications: 1) Fat people believe they must lose weight to be healthy, and 2) Skinny people think they do not need to exercise or eat well to be healthy. The reality is that eating well and exercising usually leads an individual to better health no matter their current situation.

The HAES philosophy is a simple way to approach health, with a few core principles as noted by Linda Bacon, Ph.D., a nutrition professor at City College of San Francisco and a leading advocate for the HAES approach:

- Accepting and respecting the natural diversity of body sizes and shapes.

- Eating in a flexible manner that values pleasure and honors internal cues of hunger, satiety, and appetite.

- Finding the joy in moving one's body and becoming more physically vital.

In an attempt to protect the phrase "Health at Every Size" from being used by the diet industry, the Association for Size Diversity and Health trademarked the term in the summer of 2011.

The HAES approach has been shown to improve health indicators and self-esteem. In Linda Bacon's study comparing women who dieted vs. women who practiced the HAES approach, the researchers discovered that individuals who practiced HAES maintained long-term behavioral changes, whereas individuals who used the dieting approach did not. The study also found that the "reduction in dieting behavior and heightened awareness and response to body signals resulted in improved health risk indicators for obese women."

Additionally, a few studies have been done on intuitive eating, an approach to eating that is consistent with the HAES precept of honoring internal cues. The results of one study that involved college-age girls and intuitive eating noted improved self-esteem led to intuitive eating:

> General unconditional acceptance predicted body acceptance by others, body acceptance by others predicted an emphasis on body function over appearance, body acceptance by others and an emphasis on body function predicted body appreciation, and an emphasis on body function and body appreciation predicted intuitive eating.

Many individuals who consider themselves part of the fat acceptance movement and the Fatosphere have embraced the HAES model, though there is some controversy surrounding the method. See Chapter 17: Love in Action for a discussion on some controversies surrounding the HAES philosophy.

CHAPTER 6
Is It Prejudice?

Though we continually hear how the need for everyone to be thin is a move toward health, what we see in actuality is prejudice, stigma and oppression working overtime.

I often hear people suggest that by looking at a fat body they can tell how much a person eats, how much they exercise, and what kind of person lives in that body. People prejudge fat people.

The *Oxford English Dictionary* defines prejudice as a "[p]reconceived opinion not based on reason or actual experience; bias, partiality; (now) spec. unreasoned dislike, hostility, or antagonism toward, or discrimination against, a race, sex, or other class of people." Fat prejudice, stigma and oppression abound in our culture. Entire articles and books have been written detailing fat issues as a whole, and numerous studies have been conducted detailing domination in many situations. In this chapter I bring to light only a few of the most interesting and relevant statistics.

American society as a whole has preconceived negative attitudes—in other words, prejudice—toward fat individuals based solely on their body size. In their article "Confronting and Coping with Weight Stigma" Puhl and Brownell summarize the perceptions of fat individuals:

> Negative stereotypes include perceptions that obese
> people are mean, stupid, ugly, unhappy, less competent,
> sloppy, lazy, socially isolated, and lacking in self-disci-
> pline, motivations, and personal control.

Because of the panic around childhood "obesity," children
experience a great deal of fat prejudice—often experiencing
pressure or teasing from the adults who are supposed to protect
them.

Preschool-aged children already have anti-fat bias. Those
with a caregiver who have anti-fat attitudes have higher levels
of anti-fat bias. As many as 25 percent of adolescents report
weight-based teasing by their peers throughout their adolescent
years, while 48 percent report teasing by both peers and family. "Obese" adolescents report significantly higher incidence of
teasing. "Overweight" adolescents who are teased experience a
greater risk of disordered eating thoughts and behaviors than
those who are not teased, as well as psychological problems
such as anxiety, low self-esteem, depression and anger, a study
has found. Most disturbing of all, prejudice toward fat children
and teens appears to be growing, not diminishing. A recent
study by J.C. Lumeng and others has shown that fat children
are six times more likely to be bullied than children who are
not fat.

Fat individuals also experience stigma. Erving Goffman, a
sociologist writing in the 1960s, defined stigma as "an attribute
that is deeply discrediting." K.E. Friedman, J.A. Ashmore and
K.L. Applegate say that for the fat individual, stigmatized experiences include:

> Encountering physical barriers (e.g., not being able to
> find medical equipment in an appropriate size), people
> making unflattering assumptions toward the obese in-
> dividual, being avoided, excluded, ignored because of

weight, and receiving inappropriate comments from physicians.

Finally, fat individuals experience oppression. Merriam-Webster defines oppression as "unjust or cruel exercise of authority or power." As I will show in the next few paragraphs, fat individuals are denied jobs and opportunities based on their body size alone.

Body size can affect income. Being fat can reduce a white female's net worth significantly, says J. Zagorsky in an *Economics & Human Biology* article entitled "Health and Wealth: The Late-20th Century Obesity Epidemic in the U.S." Puhl and Brownell found in 2001 that fewer "obese" employees are hired into high-level positions and fewer "obese" individuals are promoted. College students have ranked "obese" individuals as "having less leadership potential, as less likely to be successful, and as less likely to be employed than normal-weight candidates" while assigning them lower starting salaries and considering them less qualified, according to a 2008 article published in the journal *Obesity*. Interestingly, individuals with a BMI over 35 experienced higher levels of perceived mistreatment when they were of higher socioeconomic status, according to another study published in *Obesity* that year. We can see that being fat can affect individuals' opportunities in terms of both employment and wealth.

We also cannot ignore the fact that fat prejudice is tied up with classism. A fat person is more likely to be poor and lower class than their thinner counterparts, nutrition professor Paul Ernsburger writes in *The Fat Studies Reader*. Ernsberger argues that fatness actually causes poverty, saying that "intelligent fat people were far more likely to end up living in poverty than intelligent thin people."

Scholars have established that fat prejudice, stigma and oppression exist in a great quantity. This discrimination and prejudice has almost doubled between 1996 and 2006, a study by

T. Andreyeva, Puhl and Brownell found. However, our society does not see this domination as an issue, since fat people are expected to lose weight in order to overcome these concerns.

CHAPTER 7
Comparing Prejudices & the Dynamics of Prejudice

One of my primary goals in this book is to examine how oppression works. One day our society will recognize fat oppression for what it is. If we do not become aware of how oppression works and of how very deceitful it can be, domination will happen yet again, only with a new deviation that will once again justify oppression. Our society will adopt another type of oppression, perhaps out of well-meaning intentions.

I, myself, have a great deal of privilege. Though I am fat, I am white, able-bodied, educated and cisgendered. Consequently, I hesitate when speaking of other oppressions. I want to be very careful to honor and respect social justice movements that have come before fat acceptance. Since I am using hooks' ideas and she speaks from her experience as a black woman, I have found myself in a bit of a bind. In using hooks' work it can be very easy to compare fat prejudice to racism. My solution to this was to use hooks' ideas only when she is speaking of domination in general. I did not do this for my dissertation, and I consequently co-opted experiences of the African-American community, a choice I regret. I am still learning, which unfortunately involves some mistakes along the way. I have walked a very fine line with this project, and I will apologize up front for any harm I may commit in writing this work. I have tried to be aware of issues involving other social justice movements.

Comparison can take the form of the "Oppression Olympics"—the "my prejudice is worse than your prejudice game," as the *Urban Dictionary* defines it. I have done my best to avoid this type of comparison; additionally, I have tried to avoid even considering the question of whether fat prejudice may be as bad as other prejudices in order to prevent undermining of the different oppressions. Rather than looking at sexism or racism as either more or less horrific or appalling than fat prejudice, I have attempted to focus on the overall way in which oppression works, as observed by hooks.

Co-opting the language and experience of individuals in other oppressions is another way in which comparing prejudices is harmful. This challenge has proven to be more difficult. When is it co-opting and when is it learning from the experiences of others? To understand the dynamics of prejudice as a whole, we have to look at the dynamics of different oppressions for similarities and differences. Since I am using the works of bell hooks, I have had to work hard to avoid co-opting experiences of other oppressions. In the end, only individuals who experience the other types of oppression can truly tell me if I crossed the line.

Hooks has addressed the idea of comparing oppressions when considering the fact that she was commonly asked "whether being black is more important than being a woman." She argues that such questions reflect the dominant ideas. The need is actually "to eradicate the underlying cultural basis and causes of sexism and other forms of group oppression."

That being said, many individuals in the fat acceptance movement worry about offending other movements, and consequently do not take advantage of what activists in other movements have learned about oppression. I believe we need to honor and respect the individuality and unique experiences of each social justice movement. At the same time, we need to recognize that all oppressions affect all of us. If we see oppressions as too unique, we are likely to allow another oppression to exist—as we can see when progressives accept fat prejudice. As I will argue in this book, when any oppression exists, we are all affected by it.

All prejudices are horrific. We should be working to eradicate all forms of prejudice, including fat prejudice. By understanding how previously studied prejudices work, we can obtain insight into the workings of fat prejudice as well as prejudice as a whole. The idea, hooks asserts, is to see compatibility rather than opposition between all forms of prejudice. One of my fundamental goals is to argue that all forms of prejudice and oppression are unacceptable. Another benefit may be a clearer understanding of the dynamics of prejudice overall.

Connections to Other Prejudices

Personally, I think I see fat discrimination as a link in an overall chain of (in some ways) similar discrimination—racism, homophobia—and yes, misogyny. The discourses are, or can be, different, yes. But the underlying hatred... oh, I think it's all part of the same pile of steaming crap.

mara commenting on *Shapely Prose*

To start with, as this quote from mara reveals, fat prejudice is a function of old institutions and old prejudices, working as both a substitute for and an outgrowth of other forms of oppression. This aspect of fat prejudice reflects hooks' assertion that "[s]ince all forms of oppression are linked in our society because they are supported by similar institutional and social structures, one system cannot be eradicated while the others remain intact." Often called intersectionality, this idea has been defined as "a theory to analyse how social and cultural categories intertwine," according to feminist scholar Susanne Knudsen.

Considering other oppressions, sexism and racism are quite easy to connect with fat prejudice. Fillyjonk, a blogger on the now defunct *Shapely Prose*, says to add ableism and classism to the list as well. I would argue that ageism belongs on the list, also. As I demonstrate in this section, allowing fat prejudice to continue allows these other prejudices legal ways to continue in our society.

The crux comes when we consider that fat individuals have little or no legal protection from discrimination. Racism and sexism are illegal throughout the United States, while fat prejudice is legal throughout most of the country. An individual cannot legally experience discrimination for being female, a person of color, or older, though such events still happen far too often. However, legally a fat person can be fired, not hired or otherwise discriminated against based on their body size.

Fat individuals experience discrimination even when they can do the job, says Sondra Solovay, an attorney who focuses on weight-based issues, although white males seldom experience fat prejudice to the level that fat individuals who are women or people of color do. Tutuer, an obstetrician gynecologist, notes the following:

> When we are raised to believe that prejudice against those who look different is wrong, it is a relief to find a prejudice against those who look different that is right. Overt racism, sexism, ageism and even homophobia are out. Fortunately, discrimination against the overweight has never been more in.

According to Solovay, though fat individuals have some protection through the Americans with Disabilities Act, many fat people do not consider themselves disabled.

By allowing fat prejudice to continue, other forms of oppression can continue as well. Because of the legal situation, racism can still function in the guise of fat prejudice. Paul Campos argues that fat prejudice, in fact, acts as a replacement for racism.

Campos has examined the tale of Anamarie Regino, a fat Latina child who was taken from her parents even after they religiously had her follow a 550-calorie-a-day diet. Campos argues that the removal was based on racial and socioeconomic bias.

Paul Ernsberger argues that many groups, including Native Americans (i.e., indigenous peoples), blacks, Hispanics (Chicano/Chicana and Latino/Latina), and Jews, are genetically more likely to have heavier bodies. Connecting race and genetics can be problematic, however, since individuals of the same designated race may have different origins. It would be better to look at the ethnic background of individuals. Sports science researchers Dale Wagner and Vivian Heyward report that many individuals with African ancestry have heavier body structures than do whites. As a result of such differences it can be hard to define where racial prejudice ends and fat prejudice begins.

Political science professor Eric Oliver, author of *Fat Politics,* argues that fat is being used to justify social control of minorities:

> For some on the right, the obesity epidemic merely reinforces their beliefs about the cause of the ever-widening gap between the rich and poor or between whites and minorities. After all, if African Americans, Latinos, or the poor are becoming fatter than America's predominantly white elite, it is only more proof that they lack the responsibility to take care of themselves.

For ethnic groups in America, fat prejudice can be used as a replacement for racism.

Fat prejudice also can be used as a form of sexism. In other words, fat prejudice is used to justify sexist situations, to choose men over women, to judge women and find them wanting, and to control and constrain women. Campos claims that areas of the body often seen as too fat "are the areas that make (women) look like women." For more information on sexism and fat, see "Why Feminists Should Support Fat Acceptance" in this chapter.

Fat prejudice also contains very strong elements of classism. The idea that anyone has the ability to eat healthy food and exercise, if they so desire, does not take into account the situation of many individuals who live in poverty. These individuals may not have a safe place to exercise, according to a study by health researchers S.E. Parks, R.A. Housemann and R.C. Brownson. Access to healthy food is often limited in poverty stricken areas—a situation that is being called "a food desert." Additionally, many affordable foods provide high calories but low nutrition, psychologist Adam Drewnowski and nutrition researcher Nicole Darmon found, causing poor individuals to sit at the higher end of their natural weight range. Poverty thus can intensify an individual's weight, making a poor person fatter than a wealthy individual with the same physical makeup.

However, though poverty does appear to exacerbate fatness, fatness appears to cause poverty. Ernsberger declares that while "there is some evidence that poverty is fattening, there is much stronger evidence that fatness is impoverishing," a belief that is echoed by Janna Fikkan and Esther Rothblum. This pattern can be a vicious downward cycle: A fat individual cannot find adequate employment, causing lower income, which causes less access to health care and healthy foods, which causes higher weight, which causes less access to adequate employment, leaving fat individuals more likely to experience poverty.

The difference between these two causes of fatness can be quite significant. If poverty causes fatness, then a poor, fat person can be seen as once again not taking responsibility, since our society—right wingers, primarily—tends to see poverty as self-inflicted. However, if fatness causes poverty, then society must take responsibility for prejudice and domination.

Fatosphere participants have found that intersectionality has added complications to the issues surrounding fat. For instance, adding race into the mix can complicate issues of health and beauty. Linda, writer of the blog *Ample Proportions*, asserts that issues specific to Native Americans such as tribal health care create additional problems to acceptance of the HAES philosophy. The blogger Julia stated that she never really fell for the beauty ideal since "As a Woman of Color, I've felt the pain of knowing that, because of my race, I cannot be beautiful." Mean Asian Girl, a guest blogger on *Shapely Prose,* talks about the search for beauty when, because of intersectionality, the beauty ideal is unattainable:

> Those of us who are fat, or use a wheelchair, or have teeth that aren't white, or skin that isn't either, or slanted eyes, or hair where we shouldn't, or not enough hair where we should, or a variety of other characteristics or combinations thereof, would have to do a lot of erasing and adding and subtracting to reach some kind of beauty ideal. If we don't, or sometimes even if we do, at some point someone in this society will tell us we're ugly. We hear it enough and we start to believe it. That sucks, and it's hard to overcome. Despite my own efforts, I certainly haven't managed to do it. But self-hatred is a lot of work, too.

We see that ideas of beauty and health become even more complicated for individuals who experience an intersection of other social justice issues along with fat prejudice.

Intersectionality creates further complications because not only is fat prejudice a replacement for and an outgrowth of former prejudices, but other forms of prejudice add to fat prejudice:

If we're hoping to—slowly, painstakingly—help birth a more enlightened society, we have to realize how deeply these attitudes run in our current one. Fatphobia is something of a fad right now, but only because it's the latest in a long line of scapegoats; it may be trendy, but it comes from a deep-seated place. And as we try to tease it out, we have to recognize that its roots—xenophobia, parochialism, moralism, fear of the unknown—will try to anchor it. That's why fat activism has to consciously undertake intersectionality. We're not going to get anywhere just chipping away at fatphobia from above, when all the real action is under the surface. When you encounter anti-fat attitudes, think not only about how they manifest, but where they come from. We need to be ready to get at them from the root.

fillyjonk on *Shapely Prose*

As this quote from the blogger fillyjonk suggests, in order to eradicate previous forms of oppression, we must eradicate fat prejudice. As noted previously, hooks states that we must eliminate all forms of domination because they are intricately linked. We need to transform our entire culture, she says, removing all systems of domination. For more on intersectionality, see Chapter 18: Fat Acceptance for Everyone.

Liberation struggles must include the desire to end all oppressions, hooks asserts, and to do so is the only way to incite revolutionary change. We must also acknowledge the unique situation of individuals who may have additional layers of complexity because they experience more than one type of oppression:

Because each individual starts the process of engagement in feminist struggle at a unique level of awareness, very real differences in experience, perspective, and knowledge make developing varied strategies for participation and transformation a necessary agenda.

bell hooks

When we realize that our society has established much of the same situation with fat as with other social domination issues, hooks' assertions make a great deal of sense. By allowing fat prejudice to be practiced, we are actually allowing for other forms of prejudice to continue. And, most important, we are allowing the same dynamics—acceptable and unacceptable, dominated and dominating, superior and inferior—to continue.

Healthism

The kierarchy has found a way to justify prejudice—a way that gets the majority of liberals and conservatives behind this oppression (how very diabolical!). They call fat unhealthy.

For fat prejudice to work, we must first believe fat is unhealthy (see Chapter 5: The Myth of Justified Oppression for the debunking of that myth), and we must believe that society has a right to police the health of other individuals, an idea I will examine in this section. This justification of stigma exemplifies a new prejudice sneaking into our society, a prejudice so devious that many liberals have adopted it with abandon—healthism.

The term "healthism" was originated by Robert Crawford, who described it in his 1980 article "Healthism and the medicalization of everyday life."

> Healthism represents a particular way of viewing the health problem, and is characteristic of the new health consciousness and movements. It can best be understood as a form of medicalization, meaning that it still retains key medical notions. Like medicine, healthism situates the problem of health and disease at the level of the individual. Solutions are formulated at that level as well. To the extent that healthism shapes popular beliefs, we

will continue to have a non-political, and therefore, ultimately ineffective conception and strategy of health promotion. Further, by elevating health to a super value, a metaphor for all that is good in life, healthism reinforces the privatization of the struggle for generalized well-being.

Healthism, like any other of the "isms," argues that one type of person is better than another—this time based on health. Since fat is seen as unhealthy, regardless of their actual wellbeing, fat people are viewed as morally "bad."

Healthism is a form of elitism. Though some health care in the United States may be garnered from the government, good, extensive health care involves money. Lack of monetary resources results in less access to adequate health care for most poor individuals. Healthism can be particularly harmful, producing a nasty cycle—a fat individual gets a lower paying job because of their fat, which leads to poorer healthcare, which may lead to health issues, which can increase fatness.

The idea that an individual can be morally superior based on their level of health is, of course, incredibly flawed. First, it relies on a visible level of health—a false indicator of wellbeing. Second, it justifies moral ranking of individuals—never an acceptable practice in an enlightened society.

Besides, we have no obligation to be healthy—especially since society's idea of health has little to do with actual wellbeing.

Everyone deserves to be treated fairly and with respect, whether they fit an arbitrary definition of health or not. Ragen Chastain puts it in a nutshell:

> People who follow whatever you think is the correct path to health do not deserve any more respect than those who don't. Basic human respect is not reserved for humans who do what you think that they should. Health, and any measures thereof, are not a barometer by which we should judge respectability or worth. The idea that we

are all required to do whatever someone else thinks is the most healthy for us is deeply flawed. The idea of the longest life being the most important thing is flawed. We in the US have the right to life, liberty and the pursuit of happiness. We do NOT have the obligation to pursue those things by someone else's definition, and then be judged based on someone else's scale.

For more information on the rhetoric of health and fat, see my first book, *Talking Fat: Health vs. Persuasion in the War on Our Bodies*. For more information on intersectionality, see Chapter 18: Fat Acceptance for Everyone.

Why Feminists Should Support Fat Acceptance

One day as I waited outside the office of a colleague who is an acclaimed feminist and very conscious of social justice issues, I read the many cartoons adorning her door. To my amazement the collection included a cartoon of a fat woman in a bathing suit with a ruffle and the caption, "I think the ruffle helps"— a cartoon belittling fat women. I was utterly astonished for a moment. Yet I know that feminists do often thoughtlessly perpetuate fat prejudice.

The feminist movement must include the eradication of all domination, hooks believes. Feminism, she argues, means eliminating this ideology of domination "so that the self-development of people can take precedence over imperialism, economic expansion, and material desires."

As a whole, the feminist movement has been slow to acknowledge issues surrounding body oppression. In fact, in 2012 if leading edge feminist blogs such as *Jezebel* or *Feministing* posted a fat positive piece, the comments oftened include arguments over whether or not fat is changeable and unhealthy. In my interactions with feminists in my own field, though, I have found them more open than non-feminists to the idea that fat prejudice exists and should be eliminated. I have also found a great deal of ignorance regarding fat prejudice and a great deal of resistance to supporting fat liberation.

Feminists, especially, should be aware of the issues facing fat individuals, and should be supporting resistance to fat prejudice for a variety of reasons. To start with, as mentioned before, fat prejudice is being used as a legal substitute for illegal discriminatory tactics.

Fat prejudice affects women much more than men. Women are more likely to be affected by fat discrimination. Only 5 percent of men, as compared to 10 percent of women, report fat discrimination. Moreover, women experience problems in relationships as well as job discrimination at much lower weights than do men. Women start experiencing fat discrimination at a BMI of 27, while men do not until a BMI of 35, argues Rebecca Puhl and other researchers out of the Rudd Center for Food Policy & Obesity.

Men are somewhat protected from this discrimination, but women are largely unprotected, say Cheryl Maranto and Ann Stenoien. Fat women are more likely to experience poverty than are fat men, nutrition professor Paul Ernsberger maintains. A study conducted by N.H. Falkner and colleagues found that fat women are also more likely to experience mistreatment at the hands of strangers than are fat men. This trend is not surprising, since "sexist thinking about the body meant that everyone placed more value on female appearance than on the appearance of males," hooks states. Consequently, women do, indeed, experience more fat prejudice than men.

Feminist scholars such as political sociologist Gwyn Kirk, social worker Margo Okazawa-Rey and advertising expert Jean Kilbourne assert that intolerance of weight is being used to keep people, especially women, contained and constrained. This constraint becomes very evident when we look at the body styles and history of women.

As women have gained rights their bodies have been more and more controlled, feminist scholar Catherine Manton found in her book *Fed Up: Women and Food in America*. Women gained the right to vote in 1920, and shortly thereafter the flapper body style—a boyishly slim physique lacking breasts—came into fashion. As women started gaining rights in the 1960s the Twiggy style—a slim and boyish look—came in. From that time on, in fact, we see the inverse correlation, in that as women gained autonomy and power the accepted body size became smaller and smaller. Kirk and Okazawa-Rey assert that this constrained body image oppresses women and girls by "taking up time, money, and attention that could be devoted to other aspects of life, like education or self-development, or to wider issues such as the need for affordable health care, child care, elder care, and jobs with decent pay and benefits."

This "obsession with thinness is most deeply about cutting girls and women down to size," Jean Kilbourne maintains. As Naomi Wolf states in *The Beauty Myth*, "Dieting is the most potent political sedative in women's history; a quietly mad population is a tractable one."

Using a great deal of energy and resources to maintain an unattainable ideal, women are "undermined in self-confidence, mental health, and self-esteem," Eric Oliver states. The ideal body weight for women in the United States has been dropping since the early 1900s. Oliver argues that white women are pressured to conform to the severest forms of beauty standards, since they are "in the most advantageous position to challenge male power."

Fat hatred is the flip side of this thin ideal, one of the results of the United States' current obsession with thinness, Campos says. In order for thin to be the ideal, fat must be seen as unacceptable. In order to overcome our obsession with thinness, we must accept fat. Otherwise, as Marilyn Wann says, the fear of fat will always engender the cult of thinness, and women will pay the price. As the blogger fillyjonk notes, in the United States "a woman's highest goal is to disappear." Furthermore, as we shall see in a later section, when thin is a cultural obsession, fat women continually receive the message that they are in some way wrong or bad for being fat.

This cultural obsession is killing girls and women. Not only are eating disorders increasing at an alarming rate in teenage girls, but they are increasing in women and men of all ages. Up to 30 percent of adolescent girls are estimated to have disordered eating habits. One of the primary precursors to the prevalence of eating disorders is the incidence of weight loss dieting. Body dissatisfaction, not weight, increases suicide risks in girls. Simply hating fat is dangerous to young women.

Finally, as I show throughout this book, fat prejudice follows the same dynamic as every other form of oppression, as hooks' ideology of domination attests. To eliminate sexism, we must eliminate fat oppression. In fact, to eliminate any type of oppression, we must eliminate fat oppression.

The fact that many feminists buy into fat oppression in the name of health still does not make it any more acceptable than racism, sexism, or homophobia. The fact that the fat body is changeable should not make it an acceptable oppression—to feminists or to anyone else who believes in social justice. As hooks argues, if we leave any oppression intact, we will continue to have a culture of domination.

There are many reasons feminists should support fat acceptance—reasons that range from basic dignity of humans to how fat hatred affects women. Like all oppressions, fat hatred affects everyone—even those who are not fat—and should be stopped. As long as we allow fat prejudice to stand unopposed, many of the attitudes that feminists have fought to change through the years will continue to plague us. One of the goals of feminism is to end oppression overall, argues hooks as well as Kirk and Okazawa-Rey. That being the case, the feminist cause cannot allow fat prejudice to continue being accepted.

As this section reveals, fat prejudice is alive and well and even supported by feminists and progressives in our society. This oppression has been justified by myths about health and changeability. Because it is justified, fat oppression is being used to replace and extend illegal oppressions.

How do we come to accept such oppression? In the next section, I'll examine how fat prejudice wends its way into our minds and culture—a process called internalization.

CREATING & JUSTIFYING STIGMA (INTERNALIZATION)

The truth is, you can never get away from fatphobia, any more than you can ever get away from racism or classism or homophobia or ableism or any kind of institutionalized social oppression. Short of being raised in the woods with your culture dictated by bears and wolves, there is no escaping it.

Lesley Kinzel

As the words of the author of Two Whole Cakes, Lesley Kinzel, suggest, fat prejudice inundates our society as much as other social oppressions do. When considering hooks' ideology of domination in relation to the fat experience, we must consider whether or not the dynamics that hooks describes fit the fat experience.

To consider these dynamics, I examine the route by which fat individuals come to see themselves as "bad," a process that hooks calls internalization, and the forces that add to the internalization process. I also reflect on the part rhetoric plays in the experience of the fat individual in terms of internalization. I look at the connection between fat oppression and other forms of prejudice, evidence that fat individuals are seen as inferior, negative messages that reinforce the idea that fat is inferior and the end result of such negative messages—internalized fat hatred.

CHAPTER 8
Fat People as Inferior

Fat people have a triple whammy—feeling low status, being low…and then because of the anti-fat bigotry, having
lower income and less prestigious job opportunities.

LLW on *Big Fat Blog*

As this quote from blog commenter LLW reveals, fat individuals
are perceived as inferior in our society. Like people of color,
women, and those in the lower classes—populations who
historically have been, and still can be, perceived as inferior—
fat individuals are often seen as an undesirable population. As
noted in Chapter 6: Is It Prejudice?, where I provide statistics
on fat prejudice, finding evidence that fat individuals are seen
as inferior to their slimmer counterparts has proven to be an
easy task. Evidence that fat individuals are seen as inferior can
be found everywhere from school classrooms to doctors' offices,
in the media, and in daily life.

Fat individuals can feel inundated with the message that they
are inferior—that they are abnormal. From the Fatosphere,
angrygreyrainbows discusses the following:

Being excluded, alienated and treated like crap hurts, because we are human beings and don't deserve being treated less than human…we don't deserve to be treated like [caricatures] or things or whatever.

On *The Fat Nutritionist* blog commenter erin talks of the struggle to believe she deserves respect, since she has been told "because I am fat, I'm just not good enough." Patsy, a writer on *Big Fat Blog*, sums up this experience of inferiority nicely in addressing relationship issues:

Most of us here have already heard from enough sources for enough years that we are inferior in some way, we are weak-willed, self-indulgent, lazy slobs, & that we are ugly, sexless, undesirable, & should be grateful than ANYONE will look at us, regardless of how abusive & controlling that person may be or how much he/she may want to change us.

From a young age Vicky, Julie, Jane, Laura and Melissa, participants in my focus group, all received the impression that fat was to be avoided and even hated. Julie talked of hearing how awful fat was from many different sources—"from doctors, from friends, from media, from church ("The body is a temple—don't defile it by overeating!"), and so on." Jane explains her own early perceptions of fat:

I was taught that fat was bad and hateful and fat people were ugly, stupid, lazy, dirty, [disgusting]. Being fat meant having ugly clothes that didn't fit. It meant my parents fretting about me.

As we shall see, messages of inferiority come to the fat individual from many different places—the media, family members, strangers on the street, and even doctors. Negative messages also appear in the lack of options for fat individuals. These messages work together, convincing the fat individual that they are inferior for being fat.

Negative Messages in the Home

Parents can add to the belief of fat as abhorrent, instilling the concept of "fat equals bad" from a very young age. Hooks believes that this type of oppression in the home creates the feeling of powerlessness outside the home. In hooks' example, she speaks about male domination within the home opening an individual to racism or sexism outside of the home, showing that domination of any form opens an individual to dominating forces. She also says that patriarchal families are problematic:

> Patriarchal families are not safe, constructive places for the development of identities and kinship ties free of the crippling weight of domination. Patriarchy is about domination.

Coercive domination within the home also creates contradiction, as the home is supposed to be a location of "care and connection," according to hooks.

Commenters on Fatosphere blogs have found that parents often present children with the message that they must lose weight to be acceptable. Shinobi, in a post on *Shapely Prose,* talks of being forced to play sports in an attempt to lose weight. Also on *Shapely Prose,* Amanda states, "I grew up with my family hammering at me to lose weight and live longer, I internalized it, and I brutalized myself."

Parents have often encouraged and rewarded children for losing weight, if only by their attitudes. In a blog post titled "The Self-Loathing of Our Parents," Big Liberty notes that most of her intimates, with the exception of her mother, complimented her profusely when she was starving herself. Emgee talks of this in a post discussing self-loathing on *Shapely Prose:* "Trouble is, when I was skinny and they actually were nicer to me because they liked who I was when I was skinny, it only pissed me off because I was always the same person, fat or skinny."

We can only hope these parents' actions, misguided though they were, came from love. However, such actions helped internalize the belief of fat as wrong or bad.

Sometimes parents encourage their children to lose weight so the adults' parenting skills will not be questioned and they will not be judged as poor parents. As Glenn Gaesser, professor and director of the Exercise and Wellness Program and the Healthy Lifestyles Research Center at Arizona State University, notes, women are often blamed for childhood "obesity." OTM, a blog commenter on *Shapely Prose,* shares her perception of her mother's motivations:

> My mom, reacting to my misery and being very slim herself and so not really understanding the logistics of being fat, "supported" me by helping me diet, starting with the Seven Day Diet and then a nutritionist (who advised me to stop wearing pleated skirts, since they make me look fat) and on and on.
>
> I also think there was a certain element of shame in it for my mom, too. She was a single mom and we were pretty poor and we lived in an area that did not look kindly on single moms or poor folks and I think she saw my fatness as a bad reflection on her.

Blogger Living400lbs argues that society views parents with fat kids as bad parents:

> Our culture makes it plain that Good Parents[tm] don't raise Fat Kids, because Fat Kids are Officially Bad and Unhealthy and Incorrect. So parents who want to be Good Parents will feel compelled to Do Something About The Fat Kid.

Since parents, especially mothers, are often blamed for their children being fat, this action is not surprising.

Fat individuals have found that their mothers often implied or even stated that fat was a condition to be remedied. In her interview with me, Mary stated that her mother put her on a number of diets, including Weight Watchers and Jenny Craig. Blog commenter Emgee's mother put her on a grapefruit diet, while Marianne from Cali explained that her mother encouraged her to diet:

> [She] had me on every known wacky and toxic diet on the planet in elementary school. I wasn't even a fattie then. I was on the stewardess diet and on Atkins before it was Atkins. Mom just wanted me in the "slim" pants instead of the "regular." How sick is that. She used to tell me not to wear shorts because my legs were too fat.

Blogger nutrimetry explained how she ended up gaining weight as a result of the pressure of her mother:

> Similarly, before I was dragged into dieting hell, I was a size 12. I was 15 pounds out the recommended weight range for my height....After I was now a size 18, my mother presented me with a picture of when I was a size 12 for "inspiration" to lose weight because I "hadn't always been fat"; I "had once been a size 12." I was stunned that she didn't see the irony in what she was doing.

As the examples suggest, mothers can impart the message that fat is bad to their children.

Fathers can also play a part in encouraging fat individuals to feel inadequate or unacceptable. Sometimes this comes from fathers buying into cultural ideas. Blog commenter OTM noted that her father, who was a child psychologist, bought her diet books. For their Christmas present one year, blogger Big Liberty's father put his children on diets. Commenters Alyssa and Sarah B both noted that their fathers were fat, yet talked negatively about their daughter's fat, a situation Emgee expanded upon on *Shapely Prose:*

> Yup, dad never hesitated to join in on the fat-bashing, even though I got his genetics and fat-tendency. After I gained the "freshman 15" in college, he told me I looked like a "fattening hog". And he continues to tell me that "all you need to do is eat less," to which I annoyingly respond, "Now why didn't I think of that!"

In her interview with me, Anne Lutz explained that from the age of three her father started telling her that boys would not want to date her because of her fat.

As these experiences show, individuals have found that fathers' interaction with their fat children can help internalize the belief that fat is bad.

Even when parents do not make negative comments toward their children, their own negative view of fat often affects their offspring. For instance, they may have modeled disordered eating to their children. Deneensue wrote on *Fatshionista:*

> "I've had body issues since I was little. My mother was constantly worried about her weight and always going on diets. Since the age of about 8 or so (maybe even younger, I'm not quite sure) my sister and I went on diets with her."

In her interview, Mary spoke of going on diets with her mother:

> "I went on diets with my mom several times (Weight Watchers multiple times, and Jenny Craig)—starting in maybe 8th grade and going all the way through college. She is fat too and was probably the main source of my ideas about fat."

At other times, children pick up on their fathers' body issues. As Big Liberty notes the following regarding her father: "Yes, he's a self-loather. Does that mean I have to be, too?"

By modeling disordered eating and negative body images, some parents can add to their children's internalized belief that fat is a condition to be avoided.

Even though many participants in the Fatosphere received negative messages about fat from their parents, some did receive positive feedback as well. Blog commenter Fashionablenerd said her mother "told me [every day] that beauty came in ALL sizes." Commenter Lori explained that her parents did not judge her:

> I don't ever remember feeling judged by parents for my appearance. Seriously, it's bad enough that the rest of the world does it; people should at least be able to feel secure that their parents do not base their opinion of them on how they look.

Sticky commented on *Shapely Prose* that her father never said a word about her weight. So it is apparent that some fat individuals have found support at home.

Though parents are often instrumental in the formation of thoughts on fat, other family members can play a part. Blog commenters The Bald Soprano and xenu01 both said that their grandmothers tended to be a source of body shame, with xenu01 calling her grandma a "diet pusher." On *Shapely Prose,* Estrella noted that her brother often taunted her for her weight, getting her cousins involved as well. These examples provide evidence that other family members can play a role in the fat individual's internalized fat hatred as well.

As the experiences of these fat individuals attest, family support of the dominant rhetoric reinforces internalized fat hatred. Hooks points out the incredible importance of eliminating domination within the home:

> If we are unable to resist and end domination in relations where there is care, it seems totally unimaginable that we can resist and end it in other institutionalized relations

of power.

When the home front reinforces the dominant rhetoric, the individual is more likely to internalize the message of self-hatred. For fat individuals, these negative messages within help to internalize the belief that fat is bad and therefore they are bad. This assists with the creation of internalized self-hatred.

Sources Outside the Home

> It is hard to feel adequate, let alone proud of yourself, when everywhere you look, there is literally a sign saying there's something wrong with you.
>
> Kate Harding on *Shapely Prose*

Fat individuals who are lucky enough to have healthy attitudes on fat at home often face forces outside the home that reinforce the belief that the fat body is unacceptable and unworthy. These individuals experience oppression and prejudice in many different ways. These forces start during childhood and continue into adulthood. Outside messages come from intimates—family, close friends, partners—to professionals—the medical industry specifically—and complete strangers on the street. The messages can look like caring, such as a friend or a doctor expressing concern over the health costs of an individual's weight, or abuse, such as name calling or employment discrimination. These interactions reinforce the beliefs of fat individuals that they are somehow inferior and unacceptable. For example, in a post on *Shapely Prose*, sannanina eventually realized that what she experienced was not in her imagination:

> It took me years to allow myself to acknowledge that, yes, I am disadvantaged compared to thin people, not because it is inherently bad to be fat, but because society either

does not consider that my body type exists or actively discriminates against it.

Though Susan, a member of the focus group, grew up in a family where fat was not an issue, she experienced feelings of powerlessness when she entered the world:

> Once when I was in the second grade, I was punched in the stomach by an older boy I didn't know—hard enough to knock me down and knock the wind out of me. When asked why he did it, he replied simply, "I hate her because she's fat." So I learned early that the world was dangerous for fat people.

Whether it be a fiancé who will not marry a fat woman until she loses fifty pounds (Big Liberty) or boys who ask the fat girl out only because of a lost bet (University Princess and nuckingfutz), or the many other negative experiences fat people report experiencing, fat individuals can receive the message that they are unacceptable over and over from external forces.

Media Images

Perhaps one of the most powerful external forces fat individuals face is the portrayal of fat in the media. Hooks believes that television can indoctrinate the uncritical dominated mind to absorb the values of the dominant culture: "Folks look to television to learn how to think and feel about themselves." Analyzing fat in the media reveals how shows like *The Biggest Loser* and *Dance Your Ass Off* consistently supply fat individuals with the message that they must lose weight.

One of the greatest media proponents of weight loss has been Oprah Winfrey. As an African American woman who has built an incredible media empire and is often seen as the most powerful woman within the media, Oprah has been quoted as saying that weight loss was her "single greatest accomplishment." She has often focused on weight loss, though in recent years Oprah has stated that she regrets such an emphasis. Kirstie Ally is another celebrity whose weight loss battle has been chronicled in the press. She has even made a sitcom, called *Fat Actress,* about her celebrity weight loss antics. In addition to celebrities, according to Saguy and Almeling, fat characters in television or movies are often either portrayed as villains or used for comic affect, such as Rasputia in *Norbit* and Fat Bastard in the *Austin Powers* series.

As for other media representations of fat, U.K. scholar and blogger Charlotte Cooper wrote a fascinating essay on the "headless fatty" phenomenon. Cooper says that news reports, articles and other media reporting on fat, the "obesity epidemic," or similar topics are often accompanied by a picture of a fat person "seemingly photographed unawares, with their head neatly cropped out of the picture." The blogger notes that fat people are presented "as objects, as symbols, as a collective problem, as something to be talked about." She goes on to explain the implications and repercussions of such portrayal:

> [W]e are there but we have no voice, not even a mouth in a head, no brain, no thoughts or opinions. Instead we are reduced and dehumanised as symbols of cultural fear: the body, the belly, the arse, food. There's a symbolism, too, in the way that the people in these photographs have been beheaded. It's as though we have been punished for existing, our right to speak has been removed by a prurient gaze, our headless images accompany articles that assume a world without people like us would be a better world altogether.

Cooper's overall argument emphasizes the fact that fat people are often presented without character, voice or humanity. As Jean Killbourne notes in her documentary *Killing Us Softly 4,* "Turning a human being into a thing is almost always the first step toward justifying violence against that person."

Kath Read, also known as Fat Heffalump in the Fatosphere, described seeing her own body as a headless fatty:

> We recognise ourselves, even with our heads removed. I cannot tell you what it is like to be watching the evening news and to see your own body, head removed, in a story that is calling for your eradication.

> I can't tell you how devastating that is. I can tell you that later that year, after the first time I saw my own body on the evening news, I tried to take my own life. I felt so worthless because no matter what I did, I could not make myself thin, and because everywhere I turned, someone was saying that I should be eradicated. I was not a person, I was part of the "OBESITY EPIDEMIC".

As these experiences and insights reveal, fat individuals are inundated by the media with the message that they are inferior. Commenters and bloggers in the Fatosphere note that Hollywood is one of the bigger factors in the belief that fat individuals are inferior. In a discussion of Kirstie Alley's weight gain and subsequent self-attacks on the topic, Jane voiced her frustration:

> Self-loathing is not a fucking character-builder. It doesn't make you stronger. It doesn't make you better. It's just an ever-deepening, creepy-ass trap; a trap that is a huge moneymaker for corporations that do not have and never will have good intentions. You're not disgusting. You're not freakish. You're not ugly. And you're never going to be perfect. And holy shit, that is so okay.

Blog commenter Lori adds that self-loathing by fat celebrities supports the diet industry and, in fact, acts as a diet advertisement. When discussing Carnie Wilson's public weight loss and subsequent public weight gain on the blog *Shapely Prose*, vivelafat explained that public failures lead to self-blame on the part of the celebrity:

I feel for Carnie (although I am admittedly empathetic to a fault). She was told the same tripe we all were, and to "fail" so publicly at something that is supposed to be fail safe I would imagine would be very difficult. What's worse is that, without FA, Carnie has no recourse but to blame herself.

This self-blame reinforces the inferiority of fat individuals, since it reinforces the beliefs that a fat individual must change to fit society ideals and that weight-loss failure can be blamed on the fat individual.

Perhaps one of the most shining examples of fat prejudice in the media is the use of fat suits. Fat suits are used for humor (think Gwyneth Paltrow in *Shallow Hal*) or to show the origin of a character's insecurities (the character of Monica on *Friends*). One of the more damaging uses of fat suits is the oh-my-god-fat-people-experience-prejudice meme that turns up in reality TV shows such as Tyra Banks' fat suit experiment. Such experiments assume fat people are lying when they report prejudice and disrespectful behavior. Otherwise, fat individuals' experiences should be proof enough. Blogger Big Liberty argues that such experiments mock the fat experience:

> Thin people dress in fat suits not to validate the fat experience, but to mock and eliminate it. Really, I don't think there's any other reason. If they're bad-intentioned, it's to mock, if they're good-intentioned, it's to suggest costuming and playing at something is the same as being something, hence eliminating the true experience of fatness.

Though the entertainment and media industries are powerful purveyors of the "fat is bad" attitude, semi-positive and positive portrayals of fat are starting to appear in the media. *Drop Dead Diva*, a show that debuted in the summer of 2009, though still filled with stereotypical fat images such as constant eating and lack of exercise, seeks to humanize a fat woman and the struggles she faces. The premise of the show includes a "model wannabe" who, after an accidental death, returns to Earth in the body of a plus-sized attorney. According to Lifetime, "Deb must come to terms with inhabiting Jane's frame and learn to reconcile her beauty queen ways with her brilliant new mind." *Huge,* a show that debuted on ABC Family in the summer of 2010, also attempts to show fat people as people, though with a less stereotypical view than *Drop Dead Diva.* Taking place at a fat camp for teens, this show examines the issues surrounding the lives of fat teenagers "as they look beneath the surface to discover their true selves and the truth about each other," notes ABC Family.

Anansa Sims and Ashley Graham, plus-size models, have been in high demand in the modeling world. The women's magazine *Glamour* had such a positive reaction to a single photo of plus-size model Lizzie Miller in the September 2009 issue that they chose to use more images of plus-size models in the coming months. Gabourey Sidibe, one of the Best Actress Oscar nominees in 2010, is proving to be an excellent example of a fat black woman with confidence and style. Yet these plus-sized models and actresses are portrayed as a kind of exotic, sexualized oddity rather than just the natural variety of women. For instance, after the success of Lizzie Miller's single photo, *Glamour* magazine ran a photo of plus-sized models naked and piled together in suggestive poses in the November issue.

At least fat persons are starting to be portrayed in a somewhat more positive light in the media. However, this does not balance the many negative messages fat individuals receive from many different places.

Fat as Immorality

When looking at the roots of fat prejudice, we cannot ignore the moral and religious influences on the belief that fat is bad. As noted in Chapter 5: The Myth of Justified Oppression, the dominant rhetoric says all fat individuals overeat. Since one of the famous seven deadly sins is gluttony, Christianity often instills fat with a negative morality. In fact, a number of Christian weight loss programs have popped up in recent decades. Weigh Down, a "faith-based weight loss" program that calls itself a ministry, is one of the most popular of these.

For those with a white, Anglo-Saxon, Protestant background, there is a puritanical history. This history is exemplified by Victorian ideals that still can induce guilt and pleasure, especially regarding women's appetites—for sex, food, whatever—says feminist philosopher Susan Bordo.

Christianity is not the only religion that buys into the belief that a truly spiritual life leads to a thinner body. Buddhist master Thich Nhat Hanh joined with nutritionist Dr. Lilian Cheung to create a diet book named *Savor: Mindful Eating, Mindful Life*.

Members of the Fatosphere have discussed this connection between fat, eating and morality. Blog commenter Tal notes that "[w]e overindulge (sin) and then deprive ourselves (penance) in a never-ending cycle of trying to be saintly, but failing in our inherent humanity." Blogger Living400lbs suggests reasons as to why overeating is seen as a moral issue:

> Different reasons are given for why it's morally wrong, but they often include: overeating is an expression of greed; overeating prevents others from eating; overeating is wasteful; and overeating is unhealthy.

And, again, all of these ideas assume the fat person is overeating, which may or may not be the case.

Adding a moral element to fat has provided more fuel for current fat prejudice, at least within this population. If a fat person is "sinning," then it is easy to label them as bad or wrong.

The Medical Community

The problem is that doctors who see a fat person so often fail to look beyond the fat, and not only fail to see nothing but the fat, but in the process, deny treatment for whatever is actually wrong with you.

Interview with Ann K.

Fat individuals can receive the message from medical personnel that their bodies are wrong or broken, a fact that Ann K. pointed out in the quote above from her interview.

We can often find fat prejudice in medical situations. Doctors in Canada move fat patients to the bottom of the waiting list or refuse to treat them outright, N. Köhler and B. Righton have reported. Marlene Schwartz, Heather O'Neal Chambliss, Kelly Brownell, Steven Blair and Charles Billington discovered that "obesity" experts—doctors treating "obesity," "obesity" researchers, and the like—often have a strong bias against fat individuals and tend to see obese patients as "lazy, stupid and worthless." Forty percent of physicians have negative attitudes toward obese individuals, a study published in *BMC Health Services Research* found.

Negative attitudes are so prevalent in the medical field, in fact, that fat individuals often hesitate to seek medical care, according to a 1995 article in *Women's Health*. "Only drug addiction, alcoholism, and mental illness aroused more negative feelings than obesity," argue A.N. Fabricatore, T.A. Wadden and G.D. Foster in a chapter in the 2005 book *Weight Bias: Nature, Consequences, and Remedies.* At least 50 percent of primary care physicians see obese individuals as noncompliant, Fabricatore et al. revealed, while another study by Foster and crew found that primary care physicians tend to see obese individuals as "awkward, unattractive, ugly, and noncompliant." Hebl and

Xu say physicians recommend psychological counseling to obese patients significantly more often than to normal weight individuals, "suggesting a belief that those who are overweight must also be unhappy and unstable." In short, a great deal of research suggests that fat prejudice is rampant in the medical field.

Fat individuals in the Fatosphere experience so many difficult situations in dealing with the medical community that they created a blog just to discuss medical atrocities. The blog *First, Do No Harm* allows fat individuals to email stories of problems dealing with doctors, which Vesta44 then posts on the site. Story after story details everything from small incidences to life-threatening abuses fat individuals experience at the hands of doctors. Such experiences include a pediatrician who ignored all the signs of anorexia because the patient had been overweight (Kitty), to the constant suggestion to try weight-loss surgery (Christine), to taking unneeded blood-pressure medicine (Jack), to having lactose intolerance blamed on being fat (Mareen).

HappyWriter details the excruciatingly painful process of seeing doctor after doctor and being told her weight was the problem again and again, even experiencing behavior meant to humiliate and shame her into losing weight. Eventually she was diagnosed with MS by a doctor who took her symptoms seriously. She explains:

> [I've] had so much blamed on my weight, sometimes, I just prayed to get a doctor who would listen to me and see me as a person before they see the weight. I was finally diagnosed with MS, but I have to wonder—if it could've been caught earlier if I had a [doctor] who listened and [had] taken me seriously.

After a doctor at Johns Hopkins refused to remove a cancerous tumor on her kidney because of her size, Suzy Smith had to choose another doctor, which delayed her surgery by two months.

These stories detail just a few of the experiences resulting from fat prejudice by doctors that are floating around the Fatosphere, showing that fat individuals are often told that they are inferior in some way by medical professionals.

Another way fat individuals can come to believe that they are inferior is that people, especially medical personnel, often accuse them of lying about their diets and exercise. In a conversation on *The Rotund* entitled "On Disrespecting Doctors," Marshmallow told of a frustrating experience when seeking help for a foot injury. The doctor told her to eat less and exercise—that would solve the soreness in her foot. When she explained that she already exercised a great deal, the doctor interrupted her, saying, "Don't take this the wrong way, but if you really did that much exercise? You would look very different now."

Even when fat individuals are not accused of lying, their bodies are:

At my last appointment (to have a routine physical) the doctor took my blood pressure four times (it is naturally low) then said that he didn't believe the results. When I mentioned that he had taken it four times, and that the nurse had taken it three, and asked him if his office was typically incompetent at taking blood pressure he backed off.

Interview with Anne Lutz

Fat individuals can receive the message that they are not honest about their habits, therefore they are inferior.

Fat Cats and Political Prejudice

The kierarchy has done an incredibly good job justifying fat prejudice to the point that most liberals cannot imagine protection for fat individuals. Where progressives will fight tooth and nail for the rights of other oppressed groups from LGBT individuals to people of color to individuals who are disabled (as well they should), fat stigma gets the response, "But fat is unhealthy!"

The Occupy Wall Street movement is great example of liberals perpetuating fat hatred. From signs showing the exploiters as fat pigs to calling them "fat cats," fat is repeatedly the image used to vilify the rich. As Ben Spatz points out on the blog *Cacophony*, portraying the exploiter as fat is entirely wrong since "[f]atness in the United States is correlated with low incomes."

Liberals often connect fat with overconsumption. Daniel Ben-Ami examines this connection in his article "Why People Hate Fat Americans." He notes that fat is seen as the sin of gluttony, which is then associated with the sin of greed.

On the other side of the coin, conservatives often see fat as an issue of personal responsibility. For instance, in a Senate hearing Congressman Jim Sensenbrenner said regarding fat people, "The victim always finds someone else to blame for his or her own behavior."

Fat people are easy scapegoats in the political arena, since society already labels them as "Other." As Elizabeth from *Spilt Milk* says:

> In some ways fat bodies are our current culture's dumping ground for fear and loathing: we are the go-to places for thrashing out anxiety about consumption and excess, death and disease, work ethic and individual responsibility, boundaries and restraint, ugliness and beauty. Fat bodies are politicised—even politicians literally use fat

as short-hand for bad, wrong, excessive. Fat bodies are ridiculed, dehumanised, demonised and charged with meaning.

So, politically, fat individuals are attacked from all sides. All these images and messages incorrectly assume that the fat individual is fat because of overeating, a topic I have addressed before. They also assume that fat is changeable. Regardless of the situation, these negative images of fat are unacceptable.

Dealing with Others

Many fat individuals have experienced hatred in some form directed at fat, a particularly disturbing situation. Welshwmn3, a blogger at *A Day in the Fat Life*, discussed jokes involving dying fat people by noting, "People can say it's okay to kill all fat people, and that's not considered hatred? Then what is, pray tell?"

In examining the motivation behind fat hate, participants in my research suggested reasons that might explain the phenomena. Fat individuals often find that they are treated or seen as less than human or as other than human. In a response to a post written by Lesley on the *Fatshionista* blog, kdkaboom related an experience where she was described as "NOT a woman." As a guest blogger on *Shapely Prose*, Lauredhel notes that just the term "The Obese" is dehumanizing:

> The usage and context of the term "The Obese" brings home to us the fact that society thinks of fat people as a mob. A sinister, homogenised, shuffling, soulless mob. People who are fat are Othered, defined as something apart from normal. Our fatness is considered our key and defining characteristic; something that sets us apart from "regular people". Our bodies are foreign, and undesirable, and frightening. This attitude is dehumanising, deindividuating, and what's more, it gets on my wick.

Milla responded by explaining that she was called "la gorda" (the fat one) growing up in school, making her feel less than human.

In hooks' view, hateful behavior is a source of separation between the dominators and the Other; when referring to the Other, the dominated see them as subhuman. She also explains stereotypes as a way to reduce the power of the Other, making the Other less threatening. By seeing the fat individual as subhuman—whether by negating their sexual properties, using dehumanizing language, or even suggesting fat people die as a joke—society has an easier time justifying negative actions toward fat individuals.

Complete strangers often make comments regarding an individual's health, which Fatosphere bloggers call "concern trolling." Concern trolling occurs when a person acts concerned, but is really trying to shame or belittle someone. Blogger and author Lynne Murray describes it as "unsought advice and pressure from a medical professional, friend, acquaintance or total stranger using a posture of concern to supposedly 'fix' us." *Fat Heffalump* blogger Kath Read provides a nice, long list of behavior that is common to concern trolls in the Fatosphere:

- Stating that someone being fat is unhealthy—and then suggesting they kill themselves to save us all money.

- Stating that someone being fat is unhealthy—and then bitching about how much it costs the taxpayer money.

- Stating that someone being fat is unhealthy—and then diagnosing by looking at them (or a photograph of them) that they are going to explode from hernias, high blood pressure, heart attacks, arthritis and any other number of illnesses often correlated (but never causally linked to) fat.

- Shaming someone for suffering any injury or illness by pointing out that they "caused" it because they are fat.

- Stating "I'm concerned about your health!" without knowing ANYTHING about that person other than they have a fat body.

- Attributing laziness or gluttony to someone just because they have a fat body.

- Accusing someone of being irresponsible about their health because they have a fat body.

- Demanding people prove their health, or give you information about their health and wellbeing.

- Claiming people are "in denial" about their health, or their future health.

- Insisting that you know about their health better than they do.

Commenters and bloggers in the Fatosphere relate experiences of complete strangers making observations on their bodies. On *Shapely Prose*, lanalee reported receiving a comment from a complete stranger regarding her diet:

> [W]hile taking a walk, this guy at the bus stop motions for me to remove my headphones and then delivers this gem: "Fruits and vegetables! That's all you need!" I must have looked confused, because he went on to explain that "you can cheat a little with some tofu, but no meat or chips, and then I swear, it'll all drop off; it's the best diet out there." I responded that I wasn't looking for a diet, and then advised him that he didn't know me, he didn't know what I ate, and he didn't know what I wanted my body to look like, so he should keep his fucking opinions to himself.

Also on *Shapely Prose*, Becky says that it is easy to ignore such people, "but when you're fat other people make it their business." Beth summed up the fat individual's experience of body commentary by others:

> I'm so tired of my body being public property and the topic of everyone's conversation. And they think they're being nice. And they are expressing their own fears and their own lack of body acceptance and I get that. But it's my body.

Even as adults, fat individuals can experience bullying, an extreme form of outside pressure to conform. I have read of fat adults experiencing everything from teasing and catcalls to physical abuse. Ragen Chastain notes that such behavior greatly affects fat individuals:

> I think tragically, fat people hide. Not because they want to, but because they don't want to be publicly humiliated. So they don't run for city council, they don't take that class, they don't go to the gym, they don't go for their PhD to become a professor, they turn down that opportunity to speak at a local organization. Not because they don't want to do these things, but because they fear the junior high school teasing that can come along with it.

> Ragen Chastain on *Dances with Fat*

Perhaps the most horrifying element of all these external forces is the fact that many people believe that such behavior is good for a fat person because it may lead to weight loss. Fat people are shamed to lose weight, which they fail at because it doesn't work, which adds to those feelings of internalized self-hatred.

CHAPTER 9
Lack of Options

Society imparts negative messages regarding fat in subtle and overt
ways. One of the subtle ways is that fat individuals often experience a lack of options in different areas of their lives.

In one short little sentence hooks reveals the definition of
oppression—she notes that "[b]eing oppressed means the absence of choices." As an example, she explains the difference
between oppression and exploitation and discrimination of
women. She argues that patriarchy provides some women some
choices, making them forget that others are oppressed:

> Under capitalism, patriarchy is structured so that sexism
> restricts women's behavior in some realms even as freedom
> from limitations is allowed in other spheres. The absence
> of extreme restrictions leads many women to ignore
> the areas in which they are exploited or discriminated
> against; it may even lead them to imagine that no women
> are oppressed.

For oppressed individuals, this means that they have fewer
options and resources than those who exist as the privileged.
This lack of options may appear in everything from seemingly
small issues such as clothes choices to issues with more dire

consequences, such as travel.

Lack of Clothing Options

Fat individuals can feel this lack of choices when it comes to clothing options, often expressing the feeling that fewer clothes options for fat individuals acts as punishment for being fat.

We see this argument in the Fatosphere. For instance, when contemplating an idea she attributes to commenter BuffPuff, Marianne Kirby asks, "[I]f clothes are a form of self-expression and we are denied the means to express ourselves, what then?" Buffpuff herself explains that a lack of options reduces the visibility of fat individuals: "It's the visibility factor that comes back again and again to clothes for me, and the reason why the consistent lack of choice affronts me so deeply." Commenter Simply Mac bemoans the lack of plus size clothing for pregnant women, while Liz L is frustrated with the lack of plus size costumes for belly dancing. Commenter Stichtowhere says that she has actually "hermitted myself on many occasions because" of a lack of clothing options.

Kath Read explains why a lack of clothing options can affect career options for fat individuals:

> Then it came to work, and I couldn't find clothes that matched those that my professional peers were wearing. Instead, more shapeless, sloppy, dark sacks—which in turn made others (and myself) believe that I was less capable, less committed, less able than my thin peers. After all, if you can't dress yourself confidently, surely you can't do anything else confidently, right?

Even fat men experience a lack of clothing options, as Nicholas Perkins, a blogger on the Australian site *The Axis of Fat*, notes.

Kath Read explains that limiting is a form of control:

The limited options available to fat people mean that the messages we are able to send with our fashion are, in a way, censored. By refusing to cater to us, fashion labels are controlling the way we can present ourselves. (The idea that all fat women are sexless and sloppy is that much easier to perpetuate when the clothes available are sexless and sloppy.) To send an accurate message of ourselves, fat people must try harder; we have to be adventurous, resourceful and inventive.

Marginalized individuals feel the lack of choice to experiment, hooks argues, since they often find that unconventional thinking and actions "may not be recognized or valued." Given the lack of clothing options for fat people, they have less ability to express themselves through appearance, revealing their marginalization.

Lack of Travel Options

Fat individuals can also experience a lack of options when traveling. A number of airlines—Southwest, American, and United, for example—require passengers of size to buy two seats. In February 2010 director and actor Kevin Smith, a fat man, was ejected from a Southwest flight for allegedly being a safety hazard. In an editorial on *Salon,* blogger Kate Harding gave a detailed explanation of the problems with requiring a fat passenger to buy a second seat. Harding pointed out that a requirement for passengers of size to buy two seats can limit fat individuals' employment options if travel is required for employment. Harding also provided an anecdote in her own life in which her sister, who could not afford two seats to fly, drove across the country to her dying mother's side:

> But that agonizing day of asking my mother to please hang on a little longer—while she was wracked with pain beyond the reach of morphine, moaning like a wounded

animal when awake enough to communicate at all—is the first thing I always think of when the debate about whether fat people deserve affordable air travel comes up. You think of some lumbering beast who had the gall to "steal" an inch of your seat that one time. I think of a dying woman waiting for the last of her babies to say goodbye.

In response to a podcast, or "fatcast," as they call it, on fat travel by bloggers Kirby and Kinzel, Heather argued that fat individuals are the airline's scapegoats, because travel is uncomfortable for everyone.

Just the fear of being ejected from a flight prevents some fat individuals from flying, or at least makes them nervous to fly. Responding to the same fatcast, Mermama3 mentioned being "a nervous wreck" when considering a family trip to Disneyland that would require a flight on Southwest. Rachel also commented on that fatcast, stating that she was "terrified and had nightmares for weeks leading up to the flight" for a business trip. Looking at this evidence, it is apparent that fat individuals can experience a lack of options when traveling.

External forces that reinforce the idea that fat is bad can permeate the experiences of many fat individuals. Fat individuals experience the message again and again that fat is horrific and to be avoided, whether it be from medical personnel or complete strangers. Fat individuals also receive the message that they are inferior through the lack of choices available to them.

Repeatedly, fat individuals receive the message that fat is unacceptable. Fat individuals turn these negative messages toward their own fat, leading to internalized fat hatred.

Chapter 10
The Result—Internalized Fat Hatred

At 11 or so years old, I was already convinced that no one would want to love me. That no one could ever possibly like me or find me interesting or, for goodness sake, think I was pretty. At 11 or so years old, I had already completely internalized the message that not only was fat a moral failing, it guaranteed that I didn't deserve anything but scorn and mockery.

Marianne Kirby

As this quote from the author/blogger Kirby suggests, fat individuals can start believing the messages that they are bad or wrong and come to hate themselves, particularly the elements of themselves that designate their inferior status—that is, their fat. Part of the process of domination emerges as the oppressed internalize the belief of their own inferiority, hooks argues, an idea she gleaned from Paulo Freire, a Brazilian scholar who greatly influenced her. The systems in place encourage the oppressed to detest the very qualities that make them oppressed, she asserts, saying the oppressed are "self-hating." In fact, this hatred of self can be so strong, Friere asserts, that "during the initial stage of the struggle, the oppressed, instead of striving for liberation,

tend themselves to become oppressors, or 'sub-oppressors'."
Thus through all of the negative messages fat individuals can
come to despise their own and others' fat; they can come to
internalize all those messages that fat is bad.

A great deal of evidence exists supporting the fact that fat
individuals do internalize the belief that fat is bad. Considering the context of fat internalization, the fact that the dieting
industry earned $61 billion in 2011, according to Marketdata
Enterprises, certainly suggests that individuals are willing to
spend a great deal of money in an attempt to eradicate fat from
their bodies. Even fat individuals have a strong anti-fat bias,
starting at as young as three years old. Marlene Schwartz and
colleagues have provided a list of disturbing trade-offs individuals would make in order to not be fat:

> Forty-six percent of respondents reported that they would
> be willing to give up at least 1 year of life rather than be
> obese, and 15% reported that they would be willing to
> give up 10 years or more of their life. In addition, 30%
> of respondents reported that they would rather be di-
> vorced than obese, 25% reported that they would rather
> be unable to have children than be obese, 15% reported
> that they would rather be severely depressed, and 14%
> reported that they would rather be alcoholic.

This self-hate is so prevalent that children as young as five
are starting to have body image issues and as young as 12 are
having liposuction, ABC News has reported. "Overweight"
girls who internalize fat stereotypes have lower self-esteem,
"psychosocial well-being," than those who do not. This can be
very dangerous, since, as hooks attests, "underlying low self-
esteem about the body" can be a source of self-sabotage.

Internalized fat hatred becomes evident when looking at
how fat individuals in my research thought, and sometimes
still think, of themselves as well as other fat individuals. For
instance, participants in the Fatosphere have voiced self-hatred

for being fat. NotOverreacting explained that she still struggles to find worth in herself: "When I look in the mirror I see a fat person, when I look in the mirror while naked I see an ugly fat person."

Some individuals have internalized the belief that by being fat they are less than human. Wish fantasized on *Shapely Prose*, "When I'm thin, I won't be a monster anymore."

Kirby, writing as The Rotund, suggests that fat individuals "are culturally conditioned to police" themselves "way more efficiently than any outside force ever could." Self-policing leads to the belief that fat individuals deserve being treated as less than and not to "even begin to hope for something else," Kirby says.

In a blog post on *The Rotund*, Naamah notes that many fat individuals truly believe that they deserve to be treated as inferior:

> We, as fat people, are taught that we deserve pretty much whatever foul treatment we get, and that to expect better is foolhardy and pointless....For every fat person who speaks ill of a doctor or of the medical profession in general, with or without reason, there are dozens more who honestly think they deserve the poor treatment they are getting.

Fat individuals can buy into the stereotypical view of fat. In her email interview, June observed her beliefs about fat as a child:

> I, like many women in this country, grew up thinking fat was bad, and therefore fat people were bad, lazy, greedy, smelly, messy, etc.

> And I was fat, therefore I must be those things, too. Well, maybe not bad. I never quite thought I was bad, but I've long believed that I was lazy and greedy and I was terrified of being "that smelly fat girl" in my classes.

Blogger Naturally Curvy calls herself a "closeted self-hating fattie." In a post on *Shapely Prose,* Elaine expressed an ingrained sense of fat loathing:

> *SELF LOVE. I mean honestly, is it just me, or does self love feel fucking impossible??...[The] fact that [I] feel [totally] disgusting precludes self-love. [A]nd I'm not sure how to get over it. [T]he fat is disgusting thing is so ingrained in me. I think of it as an absolute truth and have no idea how to deny it.*

Considering these experiences, fat individuals—even those participating in fat accepting environments—can have a prevailing sense of self-hatred and hatred toward their own bodies.

So fat individuals experience messages that lead them to internalize the belief that fat is bad, which leads them to hate themselves. These messages come from inside the home, from parents and other family members, as well as outside the home from people who believe they are showing care—doctors, friends and complete strangers. Many of the participants in my research found that this internalized message of fat hatred, a message of self-hatred, is a very powerful force in their lives. As a consequence, this force leads them to internalize the belief that they, themselves, are inferior. These beliefs lead fat individuals to aid in their own attempts to "be normal." Fat people are not just being policed, but are tending to police themselves.

These messages, which are steeped in culture, prepare the individual to be open to accepting the domination of the thin ideal. Through these messages fat individuals come to believe that they are, in fact, inferior. Without the belief that fat is inferior, fat individuals would be less likely to buy into the belief that they should change to avoid prejudice rather than society changing. Without the internalized self-hatred, fat individuals would be less likely to accept oppression and prejudice.

In understanding the connections between fat prejudice and other socially unacceptable prejudices, we can understand how fat prejudice has come to be accepted and perpetuated by scientific and cultural messages. By understanding how domination is created, we have a better chance to combat it.

As we will see in the next section, however, fat individuals find these internalized beliefs very challenging to overcome.

RESISTANCE

[E]very day I have to wake up and prepare myself for a fight. Whether it's battling against the self-hatred I've been conditioned with, the scorns of strangers I pass on the street, medical professionals if I am sick, or even family and friends who are "only trying to help and want me to be healthy and happy."

Naturally Curvy

As this quote shows, in order to overcome dominance, fat individuals must resist. They must resist the "oppressor within" (internalization), as well as the oppressor without.

Resistance is a process that can be very challenging for the fat individual. The experiences of participants in my research divulge the powerful struggle fat people face in order to improve their self esteem, live in a fat-hating society, face everyday life, and even receive efficient health care. Resistance must be a way of life for a fat individual who wants quality of life.

When referring to resistance hooks often uses the term "decolonize," which she describes as being free from the dominant rhetoric. She states that to be decolonized "means to allow to become self-governing or independent" as well as "letting go of patterns of thought and behavior that prevent us from being self-determining." To resist, then, means working toward self-determination.

Resistance also comes about in the form of practicing critical consciousness, which hooks believes is "a process by which we reflect from that interrogative standpoint on our awareness of reality." She ties the idea of critical consciousness to rhetoric by saying that such conscious changing can come from "feminist discussion," arguing that it is "dialectical struggle" (struggle within conversation) that starts educating for critical consciousness. "Critical discussion," hooks suggests, will lead to "the transformation of the world." The following chapter provides a look into the workings of resistance in terms of the fat experience.

CHAPTER 11
Fighting the "Oppressor Within"

In order to resist the dominant rhetoric, a fat individual must first resist internalized fat hatred. Fighting internalization is the first move in the fight against oppression, hooks claims: "It is necessary to remember that it is first the potential oppressor within that we must resist—the potential victim within that we must rescue—otherwise we cannot hope for an end to domination, for liberation." This emphasis on resistance to internalization forms one of the areas that hooks adds to our understanding of the structure and dynamics of dominating rhetoric.

As noted previously, hooks argues that part of the process of domination emerges as the dominated internalize the belief in their own inferiority; in other words, as the dominated become self-hating. She believes that recovery from domination is not only possible, but desirable. "In resistance," hooks says, "the exploited, the oppressed work to expose the false reality— to reclaim and recover ourselves." She claims that a change in consciousness can lead to revolutionary change:

> True politicization—coming to critical consciousness—
> is a difficult, "trying" process, one that demands that we
> give up set ways of thinking and being, that we shift our

paradigms, that we open ourselves to the unknown, the unfamiliar. Undergoing this process, we learn what it means to struggle and in this effort we experience the dignity and integrity of being that comes with revolutionary change. If we do not change our consciousness, we cannot change our actions or demand change from others.

Oppressed individuals must change the voices and beliefs that live inside their own beings as a way to end the domination process. We do this, hooks suggests, by shifting paradigms; "we learn to talk—to listen—to hear in a new way"—once again tying such a shift to rhetoric. An individual must experience this change within in order to diminish the process of domination. This may be the hardest form of resistance, this struggle with resisting internalization.

When first approaching fat acceptance, fat individuals often experience a dichotomy, a struggle, of wanting to believe fat is acceptable yet not believing fat is acceptable. This internal conflict shows up in a number of different ways within the individuals I studied. Many found a struggle between wanting to accept themselves as they are and desiring to be slimmer. Throughout the focus group, for instance, Vicky discussed her conflicting feelings over fat. On the one hand, the NOLOSE community, a community of "fat queers and our allies, with a shared commitment to feminist, anti-oppression ideology and action, seeking to end the oppression of fat people," as defined on their website, has helped her reach a state of fat acceptance. Yet she still chose to have weight loss surgery.

Also in the focus group, Jane told of old feelings about fat and how they influence her behavior without her even realizing it, Rachel mentioned wanting to accept herself at her current weight while still wanting to be slimmer, and Nicole noted that she felt ashamed of her own fat but wanted other fat individuals to accept themselves as they were. Nicole spoke a number of times of trying to negotiate this internal conflict between thinking fat is bad and accepting fat.

Once individuals start learning about fat acceptance, they often walk through a time of wanting to diet, yet wanting to accept their own fat. In a post on how hard it is to not go back to dieting, blogger fillyjonk addresses the struggle of thinking a diet is required to be healthier vs. body acceptance, using the psychological term "cognitive dissonance."

> What we're saying is that it's possible to care about your health MORE than you care about your weight, to care about your health independent of caring about your weight—but that it takes vigilance, and that you will constantly experience cognitive dissonance when you know you're taking care of yourself but people tell you that losing weight is what you need for self-care.

This cognitive dissonance is a mental place in which the individual knows that diets do not work, but the internalization and societal pressures are so powerful that the fat individual does it anyway. Fat individuals will diet even when they know it will fail, in an attempt at self-care and for their health. In the same post, fillyjonk addresses this desire to diet when discussing how hard not-dieting proves to be. She emphasizes that a focus on health rather than weight helps with such thinking:

> Learning to trust yourself and your body, learning to trust that taking care of yourself is taking care of yourself regardless of what size you might end up, is the only way to resist that cognitive dissonance, but you have to push through it first, and (especially at the beginning) that is very very hard.

In a post on *Shapely Prose,* commenter Artemis observed this cognitive dissonance with her mother when she expressed interest in Campos's *The Obesity Myth,* yet was dieting for an upcoming wedding. Blogger Kirby wrote a post noting that even though one might be fully committed to fat acceptance, there are still days when the cognitive dissonance is present. Part of the process of resisting internalization includes this mental place of wanting to be slimmer while wanting to accept the fat body as is.

Another aspect of the process of moving toward fat pride is that individuals often experience anger toward the general belief in fat hatred and dieting, as well as at themselves for buying into those beliefs. Hooks views anger as healthy rather than pathological. Not only is it a part of the healing process, but also a "necessary aspect of resistance struggle." She notes that rage is repressed in the colonization process. Though rage can be destructive, hooks argues, it "can act as a catalyst inspiring courageous action." This rage is also the catalyst for resistance:

> Even the most subjected person has moments of rage and resentment so intense that they respond, they act against. There is an inner uprising that leads to rebellion, however short-lived. It may be only momentary but it takes place. That space within oneself where resistance is possible remains.

That view of rage and anger as a natural part of the resistance process is one that resonates with the experiences of many fat individuals.

For instance, in a post on *Shapely Prose* discussing a medical study led by German researcher Norbert Stefan that demonstrated no correlation between fat and blood pressure or cholesterol levels, a number of individuals expressed this anger. EntoAggie expressed her rage at the "pervasive hate that fills this society like a sickness" in the name of health. Redblossom noted her anger at the assumption that the health of a person can be determined by how they look: "It's like, holy fear-mongering, Batman," she said. TropicalChrome spoke of how her anger scared her:

Because for years and years I wasn't ALLOWED to

be angry that people treated me like shit because I DESERVED it. It's something I can deal with only a little bit at a time because I'm terrified that the well of anger will never run dry.

This fear of one's anger and the necessity of tapping into it is echoed in hooks' explanation of her own rage: "I understood intimately that it had the potential not only to destroy but also to construct." In a later work hooks claims that walking through pain is part of the process of healing from domination: "We know that we are in pain. And it is only through facing the pain that we will be able to make it go away."

Many fat individuals in the Fatosphere echo hooks' idea that the rage may be used to fuel resistance to domination. In fact, a number of individuals see this anger as a stage in the fat liberation journey. In a post on *Shapely Prose,* Miriam Heddy noted that the anger does get better "if you find an outlet for it that feels productive," an idea echoed by Branwyn, who argued that such rage can be used constructively to speak out against fat hatred and to change people's minds. She goes on to encourage individuals to "turn that anger (which is a form of energy) into something that goes, even a little bit, toward changing the world (or even some small corner of it)." In a post on thin people supporting fat acceptance, Jo Geek said, "The anger is a reality that must be acknowledged, respected, and resolved."

Fat individuals I researched found that though anger can be disconcerting and scary, by directing it constructively, such anger can fuel positive actions.

The "Fantasy of Being Thin"

One of the reasons fat individuals continue to diet is that they can tie a great deal of hopes and dreams into the idea that someday they will be thin. Overcoming this belief can be very challenging for some fat individuals. When looking at this desire for thinness, blogger Kate Harding proposed that this desire comes from the many ideas that fat individuals wrap up in the idea of thinness—what she calls The Fantasy of Being Thin (FoBT), a concept that has struck a chord with many people in the fat acceptance crowd.

Harding wrote the post from which this term originated for *Shapely Prose*. The post garnered 552 comments, a large number for a Fatosphere blog. Harding explains that the FoBT is a form of resisting fat acceptance "that comes from other fat people and amounts to, 'DON'T YOU TAKE MY HOPE AWAY!'" Harding observes that before she embraced fat acceptance, this fantasy, this magical thinking, dominated her life:

> [T]he Fantasy of Being Thin is not just about becoming small enough to be perceived as more acceptable. It is about becoming an entirely different person—one with far more courage, confidence, and luck than the fat you has. It's not just, "When I'm thin, I'll look good in a bathing suit"; it's "When I'm thin, I will be the kind of person who struts down the beach in a bikini, making men weep."

Telling a person that dieting does not work, Harding asserts, "[D]oesn't just mean, 'All the best evidence suggests you will be fat for the rest of your life, but that's really not a terrible thing.' It means, 'You will NEVER be the person you want to be!'"

In the same post, Meowser explained that the FoBT came from the desire to conform:

> I and the shrink yesterday were talking about the fact that if you have a shot at conforming and "fitting in," what a powerful lure it is. People want acceptance and the magic bullet that will get them acceptance. They don't want to know that there isn't one. But people like me, who will never be "normal" no matter what we look like, we know, we can stop trying and be our authentic selves.

The FoBT, then, is actually an element of normalization—the desire to be normal, to be accepted. Commenters found that this fantasy hid magical thinking about relationships (Jane, Sarah, Maya's Granny), about health (wellroundedtype2), about careers (Rachel), and about realizing dreams (Dorianne ambertides).

Commenters found that resisting this fantasy, that letting it go, was a freeing experience. MTeresa states that when she let go of the FoBT, she let go of an old view of herself: "In a sense I'm not shedding weight, I'm shedding an outdated and untrue vision of myself." For Entangled, letting go of the FoBT meant understanding that people do and will continue to judge, no matter the other individuals' size. For Maya's Granny, resisting the FoBT meant learning how to play the piano at 65. Suzanne stated that she even became healthier when she quit focusing on magical thinking. So many fat individuals have found that letting go of the FoBT freed them in some way.

Questioning this fantasy of being thin is an example of resistance supported by community within a digital environment. This posting would have much less power if so many individuals in the Fatosphere had not shared their fantasies. Because this sharing took place in a digital environment many people joined in, giving the term power and relevance.

The Ongoing Battle

Even after reaching fat acceptance, fat individuals often battle with resisting negative thoughts about their own bodies, what Jane Hirschmann and Carol Munter call "Bad Body Thoughts." Hirschmann, a psychotherapist, and Munter, a psychoanalyst, have worked for many years with women suffering from eating disorders, specifically compulsive overeating, and body dissatisfaction.

These authors argue that individuals—women, specifically—

turn most negative feelings and thoughts in the direction of their bodies. These negative thoughts, they argue, are the first thing that must change for a woman to find self-acceptance.

Individuals participating in the Fatosphere speak about fighting bad body thoughts. Angrygreyrainbows explains how easy it is to fall into body shame:

> I think a big part of it is that this culture is so chock full of body-hating BS that even those of us who make a big part of their life all about acceptance can still fall into the pit of body-shame.
>
> ...
>
> Descent into bad body thoughts is never a fun thing and it's a relief to break out. Besides...how many more amazing things can I accomplish when I'm not [funneling] this ridiculous amount of energy into body [obsession] and all that silliness. I am so tired of wasting my energy on an illusion...for compromising the quality of my life for believing lies about fat.

Once the individual becomes aware of the mechanism behind such thoughts, it is possible to resist them. I found explanations on how they resist such thinking. For instance, in her interview car explains how she fights that negative thinking about her body:

> I still have trouble. Not nearly as much, but I have days I feel terribly fat. I have days I hate every item in my wardrobe, and want to cry when I go shopping and can't find anything that makes me look good. I sometimes see pictures people have taken of me that make me feel ugly. When that happens, I know in the back of my mind that it will pass, that it's temporary. One thing I do now for it is exercise, which makes me feel powerful and healthy and functional and happy. I splurged on a good treadmill that doesn't make me scared that I'm so big I'll break it, and I know that taking the time for myself will make me feel better. Sometimes I just give in, and decide that

I'll pay closer attention to myself and what I eat and be satisfied knowing I'm doing the best I can for my body. I try to be kind to myself rather than mean, because I hate how being mean felt. I think the best way I handle it is just knowing and labeling those thoughts as not good. Even in the midst of it I can tell myself "you're being unreasonable," and even if I let myself go with it for awhile I know I'll be over it eventually.

In a post on *Shapely Prose* discussing survival techniques in a fat phobic world, Godless Heathen suggested looking at positive images of fat individuals, such as "people's photos on Fatshionista[…]while avoiding media consumption."

Dealing with internalized negative body thoughts can be very challenging for fat individuals, yet people in the Fatosphere have found ways to overcome negative thinking.

Resisting the oppressor within can be a great challenge for fat individuals. However, when fat individuals are willing to walk through the process of coming to fat acceptance, they are capable of moving beyond the internalized self-hatred. Fat individuals who do move through this process find that they experience common stages that can include: hating fat and not hating fat at the same time; the cognitive dissonance of not believing in dieting yet wanting to be slimmer; experiencing anger at the dominant system; overcoming fantastical thinking about thinness; and the return of negative body thoughts even after reaching fat acceptance.

Once a fat individual finds ways to resist internalization, however, they then must oppose external forces—specifically society and its dominant messages. In the next section, I shift my focus to look more closely at these external forces and strategies that fat individuals can use to resist them.

CHAPTER 12
Resisting External Forces

And I thought how fucking unfair it is, that even when a fat person IS living the life they want to live, when they have 'let the fat person inside out' as it were, society still tries to tell that person that actually, it's a fiction. They're not really doing all the things they think they are. They can't possibly be popular, or self-aware, or fit, it's just a figment of their, and society's, imagination.

Downside-up on *Shapely Prose*

This quote from blog commenter downside-up shows just how hard it can be for a fat person to resist the external belief that their bodies are fundamentally wrong. Added to the difficulty of resisting the internal oppressor, resisting external forces can be a frustrating, exasperating, and even treacherous situation for fat individuals. Nevertheless, succeeding at resisting the external oppressor can be an empowering and liberating experience.

"To be in the margin is to be part of the whole but outside the main body," hooks says on resisting external forces, these outside entities that seek to continue the oppression. Fat individuals are practicing many ways to resist the dominant messages, including being visible, fighting against backlash, and practicing fat activism.

Visibility as a Form of Resistance

One of the primary ways in which fat individuals resist the dominant rhetoric is by being visible, an idea that is championed by Marianne Kirby. Kirby says that just being seen in public is an act of rebellion for a fat individual. When fat individuals step out in radical ways—be it exercising in public, eating in public, going to the beach, or wearing bold accessories—it aids in normalization, Kirby notes. In response to a post of Kirby's on wearing bright colors, buttercup notes that the Fatosphere has helped her see the fat body, her own and others, as normal. Being visible "is the single most important thing we as fat individuals can do" to fight fat oppression, Kirby asserts.

The fat pride community recognizes this need for neutral and positive visibility. The Coalition of Fat Rights Activists (COFRA) created a project for this very purpose, a project they call "Dare to Show Your Face." The goal of this project, paul of *Big Fat Blog* declares, "is to show the world that we are people, first and foremost, no matter what our shapes. Fat people have voices, they have stories, they have faces." COFRA started this project as a response to the headless fatty phenomena so often presented in the news.

In a fatcast, Kirby and Kinzel talked about just how important it was to be visible. Kirby noted that "visibility normalizes things." In other words, by being visible, the fat body becomes a daily occurrence rather than an oddity, everyday life rather than "the Other," a normal human being rather than something other than human. However, there is a cost to being visible—for a fat individual, this may mean everything from cat calls to bullying. As Kirby notes:

> It's not always easy to be visible—it opens you up to commentary. Some people will respond to your

challenge by hurling insults (or even milkshakes) or catcalling or mockery. But I tend to view these instances as confirmation that I am seen.

Blogger Lesley Kinzel believes that catcalling or taunting is the price for being visible, a price that is worth it because "I never wanted to avoid life out of fear. And I'm still there, still fighting to be fearless."

Clothing as Resistance

Because being visible is a political act for a fat individual, clothing can act as a form of resistance: "[I]n my experience, being fat means your clothes are never just clothes— they're a political statement even if you don't want to make one," argues Kirby.

When discussing fat individuals covering themselves up, blogger Golda explains why having comfortable clothing is important:

> Because hiding your body sends a message to others and to yourself. It sends a message that you are uncomfortable with how you look and that your body is unacceptable. It sends the message that making yourself acceptable to other people is more important than your own needs. And I can tell you that the more you try to be acceptable to other people by ignoring what you need, the more you will feel unfulfilled, angry, self-hateful, uncomfortable, and, at least in the summer, sweaty.

Fat Heffalump argues that having fashionable clothing options makes the fat individual more a part of society:

> Having access to clothes that are fashionable and on a par with general society is both empowering and deeply emotional. Because it takes away that demarcation of being socially other, and brings fat women to a point of being able to not just dress like, but BE peers to others in society.

Along these lines, members of the Fatosphere often find that being seen exercising for the joy of it can be a form of resistance. For instance, Kirby observes that by exercising in public, fat individuals break down barriers to exercise for others:

> But when fat people are visible, in marathons and dance classes and yoga studios and anywhere else people are moving their body because it is good for them to move, we break down—a little more with each viewing—the idea that fat is a barrier to exercise.

On the same post, Kimberly found thin individuals in an exercise class were even more embarrassed than she was. Marybethorama added that she "proudly paraded my fat self through the locker room *naked*," and that "[n]ow I exercise my much larger self in public outside. Just being visible is a form of resistance for fat individuals."

Whether it be wearing eye-catching clothes or exercising in public or just being in public, some fat individuals found that they can resist the dominant rhetoric by being visible.

Fighting Against the Backlash

> I guess "nothing about us without us" doesn't apply if most people don't see you as part of a stigmatized group in the first place, right?...We're just people who voluntarily and stupidly made ourselves ugly and untouchable and marked ourselves for an early and agonizing death. We can't be believed when we write about ourselves, because we're just looking for any possible excuse not to have to give up the daily gallons of soda and bathtubs full of fries we're all psychologically addicted to[...]Most of the public discourse about us has long been taken over by cranky people on diets.
>
> Meowser on *Shapely Prose*

Fat individuals can find their attempts at resistance undermined in a number of ways. The responsibility for resistance lies with those who are oppressed, hooks asserts; the margin is a space of "radical possibility." By this belief fat people are those who should be speaking up, speaking out against their own oppression. However, fat individuals can find speaking up incredibly hard, since fat acceptance can be seen as an excuse not to lose weight, the voices of thinner fat activists are given more credence than fat activists of size, and fat individuals are often told they have no right to speak out.

Resistance as an Excuse

Fat individuals often find resistance to be very difficult, since they are often perceived as lazy and slovenly and resistance is seen as an excuse. For example, Mari Paulus, the director of Conscious Weight Loss, made the following comment in regards to the event Fat Girl Speaks: A Celebration of Size, Self and Sexuality.

> The problem with this message (for compulsive overeaters) is that hating what they are doing to themselves is a big part of the driving force for them to remain free of the addiction. The more they "accept it," the less energy they have to fight for freedom from it....[T]his is a free country and we're free to say what we want, so I'll say this: Fat people celebrating to this extreme, advocating "fat positivity," is an attempt for compulsive overeaters to try not to think about what they are doing to themselves. But in doing so, they provide an incredible disservice to those who are trying to take responsibility so they can protect their long-term health and happiness.

Thus when fat individuals do finally choose to practice body acceptance, they are given the message that they are using fat acceptance as a reason to stay fat and unhealthy.

Some of the fat individuals I spoke with gave examples of having resistance seen as an excuse to stay fat. Blog commenter Sticky, when trying to discuss the HAES approach with a friend, was told "I was in denial and compared my eating to being addicted to heroin. Then she told me Jesus says heal thyself." In a post on *Big Liberty*, Chrissy observed that her father thought that fat acceptance was about "making excuses for our weight," even though she felt that fat acceptance had motivated her to become healthier.

Being accused of using fat acceptance as an excuse is so common, in fact, that it has its own Fat Hate Bingo square. (Fat Hate Bingo is a game thought up by *Red No. 3* blogger Brian Stuart in response to "repetitive talking points that get trotted out in every single conversation about fat.")

Dealing with Logical Fallacies

When arguing that fat acceptance and the HAES approach are not valid or "good," opponents of the movement often use logical fallacies such as straw man arguments and false dichotomies. According to Merriam-Webster's online dictionary, a straw man argument is "a weak or imaginary opposition (as an argument or adversary) set up only to be easily confuted." When dealing with opposition, fat acceptance advocates often have straw man arguments posed as a fat acceptance point of view. I've heard everything from "you just want everyone to be fat" to "you want everyone to be unhealthy."

For example, in an article in the magazine *Glamour*, Jess Weiner explained how loving her body almost killed her. She explained that she didn't go to doctors for years, she didn't exercise, and she didn't pay attention to what she ate. Then she proceeded to blame the body acceptance movement for poor health outcomes. This kind of reasoning is a common argument against fat acceptance. Psychologist Lizbeth Binks explains why Weiner's account is problematic:

> [S]he was never really either self-accepting or weight-accepting. She was self-avoidant and weight (awareness)-avoidant, and for that matter, HAES avoidant. While she was bravely saying the lines, she was also NOT learning about HAES, NOT reading the studies critical of the weight-based paradigm, NOT becoming part of a FA community, NOT going to the doctor, in other words NOT doing any of the work that we all have to do get through the first challenges of the paradigm shift.

Such arguments are frustrating to deal with and almost impossible to refute except by pointing out the fallacy.

Marilyn Wann gives an example of a false dichotomy fallacy when, in a commentary in a 2011 issue of the *Journal of the American Medical Association*, scholars Lindsey Murtagh and David Ludwig argued that severely obese children should be taken away from their parents rather than subjected to bariatric surgery. As Wann pointed out in a blog post on *SF Weekly*, Ludwig makes the logical fallacy of a false dichotomy—assuming that there are only two choices.

Co-opting the Language of Fat Acceptance

The diet-medical-pharmaceutical industry is aware of the fat acceptance movement. I know this because they keep "borrowing" fat acceptance ideas and turning them into dieting ideas.

This movement is gaining momentum; more and more individuals are choosing to love and accept themselves and seek health at any size rather than continue the restrict-binge-shame-restrict cycle of eating. Seeing this, the diet industry is co-opting fat acceptance terminology and ideas of acceptance to encourage individuals to love themselves skinny. This borrowing is what paul, the originator of *Big Fat Blog*, calls "fat acceptance lite."

We see a number of examples of this in the media. For instance, a weight-loss-oriented Kellogg's commercial in early 2011 features a scale that displays positive words instead of numbers, similar to the original Yay! Scale™ invented by Marilyn Wann more than a decade earlier. In a press release issued in response to Kellogg's ad campaign, Wann congratulated Kellogg's for telling women not to focus on numbers, but added that the company "didn't go far enough. Why would they tell women the good things in life rely on the unreliable approach of 'serial' dieting?"

Another example is the fact that the dominant rhetoric has adopted the fat acceptance mantra "diets don't work." As our society sees more and more evidence that dieting does not work, as noted in Chapter 5, we see more and more twists on the concept of a diet—concepts that are rooted in words, in rhetoric. Blogger paul notes that a Weight Watchers ad campaign in 2007 co-opted fat acceptance language. On the Weight Watchers website, they proudly proclaimed, "Stop dieting. Start living. Weight Watchers works because it's not a diet." Paul calls this a backhanded compliment: "[F]at acceptance has made inroads to the point where the people on the other side of the fence need to take our message to sell anything, anymore."

As we watch fat acceptance gaining ground, the dieting industry is providing some very devious backlash. In discussing an article by Marlene Schwartz and Kelly Brownell regarding body image, one *Big Fat Blog* commenter, lauramacsd, said, "[P]eople seem to think that loving your body means losing weight so that you CAN love it...rather than accepting it how it is."

In response to this backlash, people within the fat acceptance movement are required to reconsider their expressions and language to separate themselves from the diet industry yet again. It seems to be a cycle of two steps forward and one step back for those resisting the established dominant rhetoric.

Technical communication author Amy Koerber points out this dynamic of the resistance process: "[J]ust as sense can be disrupted through individual acts of resistance, it can be put back into place through new forms of disciplinary rhetoric that aim to further restrict what is possible and permissible." So the kierarchy adopts the successful moves of the resistance groups, leaving the groups to change their own plays yet again.

In response to the Weight Watchers campaign, paul suggested a flyers campaign—distributing flyers at Weight Watchers locations or pasting them on top of their posters—that proclaimed such lines as "Diets are mean," "Live or diet," and "Diets don't work." All of the flyers proclaimed that Weight Watchers actually *is* a diet.

To combat the co-opting of language, ASDAH trademarked the term Health At Every Size. Otherwise, the term could be inappropriately used for a diet campaign. Now at least that term is protected.

This co-opting of the fat acceptance movement language is an attempt by the dominant rhetoric to reassert the previously powerful position—to once more establish the inferiority of fat individuals and to make money off of the desire to not be seen as inferior.

The Myth of Promoting "Obesity"

When fat individuals choose to love their bodies—when they do choose to accept themselves—they can be accused of promoting or glorifying "obesity." For example, the feminist blog *Jezebel* reports that musician Beth Ditto, a fat woman, has been accused of promoting "obesity." One study by physicians Davide Dragone and Luca Savorelli out of England claimed that plus-sized models promote "obesity" as well. In her infamous piece attacking *Mike and Molly*, a TV program showing a loving fat couple, journalist Maura Kelly argued that showing fat people in love promotes "obesity."

Almost every time a fat person is shown in a positive light—even exercising and being fit, as Ragen Chastain can personally attest—someone will say they are promoting "obesity." Chastain notes that "this happens almost any time a fat person is shown in the media being good at anything or having any kind of success not tied to weight loss." She argues that such statements defy the odds:

> It's insulting to my years of hard work and training, and it's insulting to your intelligence. Like it's the new V8 commercial: millions of thin people, who see the same 386,170 negative messages a year about fat people, will see one of us being successful in some way, smack their foreheads and say "I coulda been fat!"

She explains why this argument is cruel and unjust:

> Not to mention that if we follow the "logic" that putting fat people in the public eye as anything other than the confirmation of a stereotype or an ad for stomach amputation is "promoting obesity," then what we are actually saying is that fat people should never see anyone who looks like them in a positive light. We seriously believe that the best thing that we can do is make sure that fat people should never see someone who looks like them being active or successful or happy. How messed up is that? How cruel? First you tell fat people that they are all lazy, unsuccessful, and [unlovable], then you purposefully hide all the evidence to the contrary under the guise of not "promoting obesity," then you use the lack of evidence that you created to "prove" that all fat people are lazy, unsuccessful and [unlovable]. I guess the next step is to make sixty billion dollars a year selling weight loss.

So by refusing to show fat individuals in a positive light, our society is increasing the stereotypes and prejudice associated with fat.

Luckily, fat activists refuse to take this criticism to heart. They keep dancing (Ragen Chastain), they keep wearing bright fun clothes (Marianne Kirby), they keep writing professionally (Lesley Kinzel), they keep speaking up (Marilyn Wann), and they keep being visible (Kath Read). And these are just a few of the fat activists speaking up and acting out—glorifying who they are and what they can do. In the process, they show fat individuals that they don't have to sit in the corner and hide at home. Brian Stewart of the blog *Red No. 3* argues that he wants to glorify fat people:

> I want to glorify fat people who resist the shame and stigmatization. I want to praise fat people who endure all manner of injustice and keep on fighting. I want to honor the fat people who stand up and demand respect. Fat people are awesome. Fat people kick ass. Fat people deserve glory. We just don't think anyone else needs to be disgraced or shamed for us to be glorified.

Thin Voices

Because of this backlash against some fat individuals who speak out, it is not surprising that many of the most prominent of authors and authorities in the fat studies movement are individuals who are not considered fat—Paul Campos, J. Eric Oliver, Glenn Gaesser, Linda Bacon and Abigail Saguy come immediately to mind—in addition to being all white, with the exception of Campos.

Thinner scholars within fat studies find that their research is more likely to be taken seriously. Paul Campos, in a talk at UCLA, said that he could talk about the "obesity" myth without ridicule because he is a man and he is socially not "overweight," even though his BMI places him in the "overweight" category. He said a woman would have more issue speaking with the same BMI. In an email conversation, Linda Bacon noted her experience with this trend:

> I'm also thin (or at least not fat). In the conventional media my words about fat acceptance unfortunately seem to carry a lot of meaning compared to my fat compatriots....I've heard frequently from fat and thin people that they are more likely to trust my words about nutrition and other issues than a fat person's. Even within the fat community, I am granted privilege....There seems to me to be more desperation among fat folks to have thin allies, than is true for other stigmatized groups.

This tendency is so strong, in fact, that many thin scholars who are exploring fat issues find their research privileged over fat studies scholars who have actually experienced fat prejudice.

Fat allies find that they have more credibility regarding fat prejudice than fat people themselves. In a guest post on *Shapely Prose*, volcanista states that she has "automatic credibility on the subject of fat prejudice, despite never having experienced it firsthand, while actual fat people are just wrong/deluded/lying. THAT makes sense."

Because of this type of thinking, fat people are usually excluded from any kind of policy proceedings regarding "obesity." Charlotte Cooper often proclaims the cry of "nothing about us without us," procured from the disability movement. This cry means that fat individuals should be integral in the making of policy on fat bodies, since they are the ones affected. Cooper notes that "obesity" conferences seldom have fat individuals represented, and how problematic this is:

> Can you imagine a conference about disability where disabled people were not central to the proceedings? Or a gathering about race or sexuality where minority ethnic or queer people were required to sit in the audience and listen politely whilst a bunch of white or straight experts told them that their lives were worthless? It would not only be insulting and patronising but also ludicrous. I'm not saying that such events don't exist, unfortunately they probably do, but they are likely to be regarded as

unsuccessful and profoundly flawed. Not so in the world of the obesity expert!

As a result of the belief that fat people could become smaller if they so choose, fat voices are muted when they speak out. Thinner individuals are given more of a creditable voice in terms of the fat experience than fat individuals themselves.

Along with the accusation of fat acceptance as an excuse not to lose weight, fat individuals often are told that they have no right to portray their own experience. As Ragen Chastain states:

> That got me thinking about how often we are told that, as fat people, everyone is a better witness to our experience than we are. We are told that we're not competent witnesses to what and how much we do or should eat, or how much we do or should exercise. Our bodies are held up as proof that we must be lying or deluded and that we can't possibly know, or be doing, what's best for us. We embrace our health and we are told that it's impossible for us to be healthy. We are told that everyone from Dr. Phil to Dr. Oz to random people on the internet know more about how we think and act than we do.

Kath Read believes that such denial of the fat individual's experience reinforces the fat person as Other:

> The other main outcome of this kind of behaviour is the othering of fat people. It reduces fat people to subnormal beings, as less-than-human others, as though they are animals that require husbandry, a kind of domestic management. It strips fat people of the fundamental human right to advocate for themselves and make their own life decisions.

So by viewing fat acceptance as an excuse not to get thin and by denying the fat person a voice, the dominant rhetoric reinforces fat oppression, undermining resistance to fat prejudice.

Living in a fat phobic culture while choosing to resist the dominant rhetoric can be a daunting task for the fat individual. However, many fat individuals have found ways of resisting the belief that they are inferior—survival techniques, if you will. These survival techniques keep fat people from buying into the belief that they are wrong or broken for being fat. Whether it is reading Fatosphere blogs, learning how to talk with parents, knowing ways of dealing with doctors, or just learning to laugh about it, fat individuals are continually finding ways of resisting the dominant messages saying fat is bad.

Fat Activism

Fat individuals can resist fat prejudice by practicing fat activism. What exactly entails fat activism, however, seems to be unclear, as revealed in both the Fatosphere and the interviews I conducted.

For example, in her interview happyhedonist notes that she isn't an activist because "[a]ll I do is refute the junk science and hateful bullshit attitudes when it comes up in conversation." Yet Finley does consider herself an activist "in a limited way," because she tries "to increase awareness of fat issues among my friends and family and encourage them to accept their bodies as they are." Anna F. does not consider herself an activist, though she will talk about fat acceptance if the subject comes up. Mustardseed did the same, but felt like the term "activist" was "putting it too strongly." Sara did not know if she was an activist, though she would speak out against dieting and weight loss. Jeanne, who does speak up at injustice and also communicates with stores and manufacturers about fat fashion, asked "Can you be a passive activist?" Andromeda argues that whether she is an activist depends on what the term means:

If you mean participating in protests and fundraisers

to get the word out there, or even writing letters to the editor, then no. However, if you mean championing the point of view that fat people deserve to be treated like everyone else and given equal rights, and not shying away from expressing this point of view to dissenters I encounter, then yes, I am.

Blogger fillyjonk notes that there exists a disagreement on what exactly fat activism means, "both what it should mean for the community, and what it means for us personally," yet speaking up for one's self is important in any situation. She goes on to give a list of examples of fat activism she has witnessed:

> Some people are awesome in-your-face street activists who never pass up a teachable moment. Some people write—for blogs and newspapers, for experienced activists and brand-new 101ers. Some people organize; others are activist through art...or radical visibility. Some people will drink a bowl of gravy for fat acceptance. Not everyone wants to speak up every time—and even when we're speaking up, we may disagree on tone and approach, honey versus vinegar.

For those who are more vocal on fat acceptance, blogger paul with the help of commenters on *Big Fat Blog* put together a media guide for bloggers who wanted to be outspoken activists.

At times, these different views on activism have caused issues within the fat acceptance communities. For instance, Stacy Bias wrote an article arguing for different types of activism. Within the article she noted that some fat activists were critical of other activists, a disheartening behavior:

> What matters is that we attempt to provide an entrance into that hallway for EVERYONE and this cannot be accomplished within the expectation that all entrants to said hallway immediately understand all the complex interweavings of oppression at play in the creation and

maintenance of the fat hatred that they may not even have considered might exist in the first place.

In other words, fat activism has many different flavors, all of which have merit. Although they have different views on what counts as activism, fat individuals are resisting the dominant rhetoric in a variety of ways.

Activism "does not need to be some kind of organized 'against' protest," hooks agrees. In fact, she argues that a person should focus on "[their] own reality" first. Otherwise, she argues, "When you're fucked-up and you lead the revolution, you are probably going to get a pretty fucked-up revolution."

In my own opinion, anytime someone speaks up for fat people, a fat person denies the kierarchy's view of fat, or a person takes a loving action toward a fat individual, it can be called activism. And every little bit of that activism is important.

Kath Read, the Fat Heffalump, explains why she is an activist:

My only way of coping is to take it on and try to change the world. I did 35 years of trying to change me to fit the world, and it didn't work—it almost killed me. Now I intend to devote the rest of my life to changing the world to fit everyone. After all, the world is a big diverse place, there is room in it for all of us, no matter who we are, what we look like or what our lives are. And we fat people have as much right to it as anyone else.

Individuals in the fat acceptance movement continue to resist the dominant rhetoric, but they continue to find it a daunting and wearying task. Though it is not clear exactly what makes a fat activist, this section can give us an idea of the actions fat activists take.

Fat activists speak out against body shaming and fat hatred while continuing to fight the message that the fat body must be changed to be loved. A fat activist may choose to be visible, and, even when being told that fat acceptance is an excuse or when thin allies are given more credence than they, they continue to speak out and step up. If nothing else, we can see a fat activist as someone who rejects the dominant rhetoric and takes steps to fight the belief that fat is bad and unacceptable.

Perseverance

> Sometimes, talking about fat acceptance feels like I'm trying to empty out Lake Michigan with a teaspoon. I really need a bigger spoon.
>
> Welshwmn3

Even with the strides they have made in their own lives, members of the fat acceptance movement admit frustration in changing such tenacious attitudes like anti-fat bias and the dieting mentality in society, as welshwmn3's quote suggests.

Fat individuals I studied voiced frustration at just how big a problem fat prejudice proved to be. When interviewed, Athena wondered if fighting body shaming was a losing battle: "I think that fat shaming is so internalised that loads [of] us are dieting even when talking up body acceptance." Athena also stated that body shame is actually increasing in power, and overcoming it is challenging: "It's such bloody hard work sometimes."

The battle to resist the dominant messages does appear daunting for fat individuals. Sometimes these changes take awhile to become evident. Fat studies author Linda Bacon discusses this in her essay on thin privilege:

> But another lesson I've learned over time is that resistance isn't valuable only when it sparks an immediate and visible change. The power of resistance is to create a safe zone—even if it's just for a moment—where fat-phobia isn't tolerated, to set an example. You may not necessarily

change the other, but you plant a seed. I can't tell you how many times people have told me over the years that they heard this message once, but it wasn't until years later that some other event catalyzed a new awareness. Without those earlier seeds, the later events wouldn't have had their impact.

Even though the dominant rhetoric has an incredible amount of power, fat individuals speak out anyway. If nothing else, they have created a safe zone—a diet-talk- and fat-hatred-free zone where all bodies are accepted. They also continue to live a life of resistance. One *Big Fat Blog* commenter considers this an act of rebellion:

> Sleeping for 8 hours a night is not only good for you, it's an act of rebellion. Working 40 reasonable hours a week (or LESS!), likewise. Wearing comfortable shoes that permit you to think productively. WOOF! Eating satisfying amounts of the foods you like. Exercising for the joy of it. REBELLION.
>
> DebraSY on *Big Fat Blog*

It may be a long road, but this resistance movement is making a difference, if only in the lives of fat individuals participating in fat acceptance and the Fatosphere.

In my opinion, the number one attribute required for a fat activist to be a success is perseverance. Whether it be advocacy or teaching or writing or whatever, sticking to it is the most important action I can take on days when I feel like I am beating my head against the wall. I have to remind myself that I make a difference. I have to remember that success is relative and that failure only comes from quitting. I get frustrated some days when I feel like the world is unchangeable. Then I will find proof that together fat activists are changing the world one reader at a time. Perseverance is a requirement for the fat activist.

CHAPTER 13
The Power of Rhetoric

There are many ways to change the world. One of them is through language. That's why groups reclaim former slurs—to reclaim the word changes the power of that word, repurposes it and changes the world.

I don't talk about my body in terms of flaws. Even if I weren't into fat/body/size/whatever flavor you call it acceptance, I wouldn't because to define things in terms of negative qualities is to define something as negative. I just don't have time for that kind of crap. I have too many other things to do to spend my mental and emotional energy in considering my body to be a negative Thing, a flawed object, a no-good construction that is somehow separate from my self.

Marianne Kirby

Another way fat individuals are changing their own and others' per-ceptions of fat is by changing their language. As the quote above from blogger Marianne Kirby illustrates, changing how the fat body is discussed changes perceptions of the fat body.

When looking at the transformation of "consciousness and being" an oppressed individual goes through when choosing to resist the dominant rhetoric, hooks maintains that language plays an important part in the effort—that we are rooted in words, that oppressed individuals must create a shared language, and that such a transformation requires a paradigm shift, a new way "to talk—to listen—to hear."

"Language is also a place of struggle," hooks says, urging the oppressed "to recover ourselves—to rewrite, to reconcile, to renew." She notes that words in themselves perform as a resistant act, and asserts that in order to resist the oppressors, the oppressed must learn a new way to speak:

> The most important of our work—the work of liberation—demands of us that we make a new language, that we create the oppositional discourse, the liberatory voice. Fundamentally, the oppressed person who has moved from object to subject speaks to us in a new way.

The individual must establish "the liberatory voice" and no longer define their status as oppressed. Fat individuals, therefore, must find a new way of talking about their bodies and the condition of being fat. By changing how they talk about their bodies, fat individuals perform an act of resistance in and of itself.

Language as resistance takes on two different aspects: how individuals within the fat acceptance communities talk among themselves, as well as how fat individuals talk to those spouting the dominant rhetoric. Through debate on blogs and discussion groups individuals within fat acceptance have created a lexicon specific to their experiences, which allows them to relate to each other, to redefine their own experiences, and to resist the external rhetoric reinforcing previous beliefs of the inferiority of the fat body. As hooks explains, this often happens with oppressed groups:

> Within any situation of colonization, of domination, the oppressed, the exploited develop various styles of relating, talking one way to one another, talking another way to those who have power to oppress and dominate, talking

in a way that allows one to be understood by someone who does not know your way of speaking, your language.

My research reveals that individuals within the fat acceptance movement have used language to resist the dominant rhetoric by redefining terms for themselves, reclaiming the word "fat," coming out of "the fat closet," resisting medical rhetoric, and employing humor. In response to these rhetorical strategies that are proving to be effective, the Fatosphere and fat acceptance movements are seeing their language co-opted—a situation they address as well. Yet, as I demonstrate in the paragraphs below, fat individuals persist in using these strategies in an effort to find their "liberatory voice."

Redefining Terms

I found that members of fat acceptance and the Fatosphere together have redefined terms, most especially those associated with health and medicine, in order to resist the dominant messages. In *The Medicalization of Society,* sociologist Peter Conrad notes that defining medical norms is "in itself a cultural form of social control, in that it creates new expectations for bodies, behavior, and health" and leads to medical expectations that "set the boundaries for behavior and well-being as well has how medical norms guide behavior." Rhetor Elizabeth Britt follows this same line of thinking by noting that definition has the power "to frame experience" and that defining terms is a vital part of normalization.

The exploited must find their own standards and truths, hooks argues; oppressed individuals must "work to expose the false reality—to reclaim and recover ourselves" for resistance to be effective. She believes that oppressed groups can redefine values, can decide how much they will compromise:

Even in the face of powerful structures of domination, it

remains possible for each of us, especially those of us who are members of oppressed and/or exploited groups...to define and determine alternative standards, to decide on the nature and extent of compromise.

By redefining terms and coming to their own understanding of what terms mean, members of the fat acceptance community undermine the dominant rhetoric, once again finding the "liberatory voice."

By establishing medical definitions of acceptable body size (see the book *Talking Fat* for an in-depth discussion of the words "normal," "overweight" and "obese"), the medical establishment creates social control. The social control implied by these definitions is exemplified by one of the sizes being labeled "normal." Using the word "normal" implies that the standard weight of the American population falls into this category, when actually only a small percentage—only 31.6 percent according to the National Institute of Diabetes and Digestive and Kidney Diseases—actually does. Marilyn Wann, in the foreword to *The Fat Studies Reader,* notes that such labels as "overweight" and "obese" medicalize human diversity and "are neither neutral nor benign."

On a discussion on "Fat Semantics" on *The Rotund,* commenter Halle says that she is offended by medical terminology, especially the word "overweight": "Over what weight? Whose weight chart? I could rant for hours about that." Blogger *Red No. 3* notes that the term "overweight" "defines us not by what we are, but by what we have failed to be."

Wann states that "overweight" "implies an extreme goal: instead of a bell curve distribution of human weights, it calls for a lone, towering, unlikely bar graph with everyone occupying the same (thin) weights."

Instead of using medical terms, members of the Fatosphere have adopted their own terms for body size. "Inbetweenies," a term that seems to have originated in the *Fatshionista* community and is therefore associated with clothing size, are those individuals that fall between acceptably skinny and very fat, usually women between American sizes 12 and 18. They can still buy clothes in the average stores and are on the low end of sizes available in plus-size stores. Members of the Fatosphere call larger individuals, usually over American size 20, "death-fat," a term which originated with Lesley at *Fatshionista*. She explains the term:

> I am super duper really for real maaaaad fat. I am the kind of fat where doctors are friendly until they get me on a scale, and then after that they get Very Somber and talk to me Seriously about my Weight Problem (which is why I no longer get on said scale at the doctor's office). I am the kind of fat where I can't always find stuff to fit me even in plus-size shops. I am the kind of fat a lot of people mean when they say, well, some people are just bigger, but people who are really fat are just not normal or healthy, and maybe those people SHOULD lose some weight. Those people are talking about me.

Lesley explains that she took the name from the medical term "morbidly obese," which the medical establishment defines as being in excess of a hundred pounds or 100 percent over maximum recommended weight.

By refusing to accept the labeling of their bodies, fat individuals therefore resist the dominant rhetoric. They also can claim fat bodies are simply a manifestation of human diversity by reclaiming the word "fat," as I will explain in a later section.

Fat individuals can also resist the dominant rhetoric through redefining the term "health," another important word in my research. The World Health Organization (WHO) defines health as "a state of complete physical, mental and social well-being and not merely the absence of disease or infirmity." The American Medical Association's policy defines it as "a state of physical and mental well-being." On the other side, many individuals in the fat acceptance movement, including Kirby, resist defining health broadly and believe that each individual should determine what health means to them.

"Health," author Marilyn Wann asserts, "can be used to police body conformity and can be code for weight-related judgments that are socially, not scientifically driven." She also believes that the current idea of health reinforces "social control around [weight] and can be very damaging to well-being."

Blogger Michelle, *The Fat Nutritionist,* discusses her own issues with the WHO definition of health, noting that it creates a controlling culture:

> It's the silent assumption that anyone experiencing less than 'ideal' health is not only possibly to blame for their predicament, but that their lives are tainted, somehow broken, and possibly less meaningful than the lives of the 'healthy.'
>
> I propose that our definition of health should have less to do with how sick or well we are, and more to do with how we live inside and with our unique physical condition.
>
> A person's state of health is what it is, and the thing to strive for is not less disease, or even longer life, but *the ability to inhabit, accept, and cope with what is.*
>
> Are we banishing disease and improving quality of life, or are we blindly, almost compulsively, seeking to bring people in line with powerful, if latent, cultural ideals?

Michelle's ideas of health take the morality and control out of the concept of health. Blogger Kate Harding also argues that health can be seen individually, that it should be defined "according to an individual's own body and its limitations."

By changing their perceptions of the word "health," fat individuals seek to resist societal control; they seek to resist the dominant rhetoric.

Another way that fat individuals can resist the dominant rhetoric is through members of the fat acceptance movement reclaiming the word "fat." This resistance to the dominant language—a resistance of words—became apparent through conversations regarding the word "fat." Though "fat" is not a new word, by changing how they speak of it fat individuals can change the way they perceive fat.

Before choosing to resist the idea that fat is inferior, a number of the participants in my research saw the word "fat" as a weapon hurled at them. In the focus group, Vicky explained the power of "the f-word":

> The word 'fat' was barely in my vocabulary. Neither were the words obese, overweight, overeat, compulsive, heavy, big. I avoided those words because they felt like weapons. They only served to hurt me. Thrown about carelessly in conversation. An accidental shooting. I felt gravely wounded when those words reached my ears. Whether I said them or heard them—whether they were about me or intended for me was irrelevant. I'd wished I could have kept my fatness a secret for the rest of my life. As if it [were] possible.

Many of the other focus group participants used to feel the same way about the word "fat." Julie, Melissa and Nicole all spoke of being afraid of the word until they learned to rebel against it. Melissa and Nicole both said they had been afraid of the word, but now choose to see it as harmless, "as just an adjective." Julie claimed a bit stronger transformation. She now sees the word as empowering: "Now, I am loud and proud in uttering the f-word and in drawing attention to my fat body and the many needs it has that are *not* fulfilled in this fat-hating culture." Until she found "the words to reclaim her body," Julie felt like she "existed only in the negative, only in the visual shadows."

Individuals in the Fatosphere have also embraced the word

"fat." Blogger Harding talks of seeing the word as a "value-neutral adjective" rather than "a terrible thing." When discussing the euphemism "fluffy" as a replacement for the word "fat," blogger Btsu says on *The Rotund:*

> Fat is substance, though. It has weight and presence. I know [it's] a tall order, but I don't want people to run from that. We aren't [helium] balloons. We have space and that's a good thing.

In a conversation on a manifesto for fat acceptance, members of *Big Fat Blog* debated using the word "fat." Cleis noted that it was "important to include and reclaim the word 'fat' as positive, affirming, and joyous." Paul concurred in the same post, saying, "That word needs to belong to us again; it needs to drop its negative connotation and the best way to do that is to combat ignorance." Again on *Big Fat Blog,* turtlegurl continues on to say:

> It is not a dirty word, it is just a three-letter adjective, & no more evil than 'tall' or 'short' or 'blonde', etc. We need to own it & speak it proudly until it stops being more shocking than the other 'f' word ever thought of being.

Individuals within the fat acceptance movement have decided to reclaim a word that had been used to hurt and attack them previously. By reclaiming a single word, fat individuals in the fat acceptance movement use language to resist the dominant rhetoric.

Part of reclaiming the word fat is considering the connotations associated with the word. Before fat acceptance, participants in the Fatosphere, including spoonfork38, found the word associated with "stupid, smelly, dirty, and ugly." Blogger *Red No. 3* explained how changing the connotation of the word is important for fat acceptance:

At its heart, fat is really just an adjective. A description. [It's] neutral on its own. Negative connotations are introduced to the word rather than being inherent in it. Fat is just fat and [it's] a word we have to reclaim. As long as "fat" is unspeakable, then fat people will be dehumanized and stigmatized. We need to make the word neutral again. We need to win it back from those who'd rather use the word as a club to beat us with than a word to describe us.

"[T]he word is so loaded in our society that it can't be a simple anything," Kirby said, noting that she rejects any negative associations with the word.

So members of the Fatosphere are attempting to change the connotations of the word to be more neutral or even positive. Yet as a whole the fat acceptance movement did not choose to embrace the word "fat" immediately.

The conversation surrounding what to call the movement was illustrated by the discussion on *Big Fat Blog* considering a manifesto for fat acceptance. Commenter Micdee69 suggested "size acceptance" instead of "fat acceptance" because the word "covers all sizes. [It's] all about personal body image and how one [perceives] oneself." However, commenters responded by claiming that "size acceptance" would not work. "Size Acceptance is OK and great," said commenter William, writing as shryve, "but I do not really see any 'Size' hate out there that compares to the Fat Hatred." Blogger paul responded with, "It's my personal belief that one can't have size acceptance as a movement until fat acceptance happens." Today, even though most fat studies scholars and fat acceptance bloggers advocate accepting people of all sizes as part of natural human diversity, "fat acceptance" is the term most often heard in the Fatosphere and within fat studies.

In hooks' view, these individuals are resisting domination through language. By changing their perceptions of a single little three-letter word, fat individuals speak out against the oppressive ideals they face in this culture. In fact, as Abigail Saguy notes, using the word "fat" often signifies an individual who has come "out" as fat—an idea we will explore in the next section.

Coming Out as Fat Accepting

One very interesting phrase that popped up often in this research illustrates another change of perception: Members of fat liberation community talk about coming out of the "fat closet," "coming out as fat," or "coming out as fat accepting." This term can be seen as problematic since, as Ruth Ginzberg said in a discussion on the Fat Studies listserv, borrowing from others is always problematic:

> I think [it's] always potentially problematic when one marginalized/oppressed group starts using language or metaphors (sometimes very hard-fought-for language, metaphor or imagery) that some other oppressed or marginalized group has fought to make meaningful to themselves. It can also be problematic if viewed as a form of comparing (or some might think, co-opting) oppressions.

By borrowing the term, the fat individual may be assuming that they understand the experience of an individual in the LGBT movement. In fact, a gay man I know became very upset when he read about this topic in my dissertation. He saw it as a way for fat individuals to co-opt the LGBT experience.

I think this statement becomes less problematic when recognizing that when fat individuals say "coming out as fat," they appear to mean "coming out as fat accepting." Everyone can see the fat, so acknowledging having a fat body is not surprising. However, fat individuals who choose to *accept* their fat is another story.

The consensus on the Fat Studies listserv appears to be that although the term "the fat closet" is problematic in a number of ways, the idea of "coming out" is an accurate reflection of the fat resistance experience. A number of fat studies scholars have used this phrase, including Kathleen LeBesco, Marilyn Wann and Abigail Saguy. In an article, Saguy argued that "coming out as fat" is a refusal to "cover." Goffman defines "covering" as withdrawing "covert attention from the stigma." Law professor Kenji Yoshino calls refusing to cover "flaunting."

Saguy suggests that the narrative of coming out may have migrated based on two possible functions. First, there is a great deal of overlap between the queer and fat acceptance movements—fat acceptance has a significant queer population, according to LeBesco. A second option may simply be the cultural assimilation of the term, according to Saguy. As Yoshino noted, "[W]e all have secret selves." Saguy suggests that it is actually those with a form of an attachment to the queer community—"residents of San Francisco…queer-identified activists, and queer theorists"—who "were among the first to talk of coming out as fat."

Obviously, fat individuals cannot hide their fat like gay people may be able to hide their sexual orientation. Rather, "coming out of the fat closet" appears to mean changing the way fat individuals talk and perceive fat and themselves.

Saguy proposed a few different aspects of coming out as fat. She noted that it involves "revealing a hidden self identification" as well as "a person who is easily recognized as fat affirming to herself and others her fatness as a nonnegotiable part aspect of self, rather than a temporary state to be remedied through weight loss." Additionally, the fat individual who is "out" rejects "cultural attitudes that fatness is unhealthy, immoral, ugly, or otherwise undesirable" and "claims the right to define the meaning of one's own body and to stake out new cultural meanings and practices around body size."

When a fat person "comes out as fat," they are saying that

they refuse to play by the rules of society regarding fat.

To members of the Fatosphere, as well as participants in the focus group, coming out as fat accepting appears to mean to quit dieting, to accept themselves as fat without self hatred, to even like and love their fat. In a post on *The Rotund,* On Reserve explains that it means to "let someone know that I'm about 99% ok with being fat." Commenters to the same post talked of coming out as fat as meaning that they are "happy with their size" (Becky) or that they do not consider fat a moral failing (Kate217).

In the focus group, a few of the participants also talked about coming out of the "fat closet." Julie said it is a bad metaphor, "but to some extent it feels right, since my body size was often in everyone's foreground but never mentioned." She also stated that fat was "the dirty little secret that everyone knew but no one mentioned." Susan said being out is a form of truth, while the current beliefs on fat health and fat beauty were the "big fat lie." Jane noted that being in the fat closet meant "not ever talking about it to anyone and living in fear that someone would mention that I was fat."

So coming out as fat accepting means things like the "right to live in and love my body" (Julie) and going public about "considering myself fat" (Ann). To come out as fat means changing the way fat individuals talk and perceive fat and themselves. It means finding that "liberatory voice."

Resistance to Medical Rhetoric

Another area in which fat individuals practice survival techniques is in the medical field, where many have found that resistance is required when dealing with the medical industry in order to obtain good health care. For instance, fat individuals often "get a diet, rather than a diagnosis" when dealing with the medical community, Wann notes.

In her interview, car expressed frustration at doctors' stubborn refusal to accept the scientific evidence that fat does not immediately equal a health risk. "The 'easy' answer is still that fat is bad and unhealthy," she said, "and it seems that stories that show it's not that simple are just buried."

In order to resist fat bias, fat individuals must learn to transverse cultural, medical and scientific rhetoric—often learning to formulate science-based arguments just to receive basic necessities like health care. In a post on *Shapely Prose*, Piper argues on "how important it is as a fat person to arm yourself with knowledge" when dealing with doctors.

Fat individuals have a number of different techniques that assist them in resisting the dominant rhetoric when dealing with health care situations.

A common technique used by some individuals in the Fatosphere is sending a letter to a new doctor. The text of this letter can be borrowed from Hanne Blank (http://cat-and-dragon.com/stef/fat/hanne.html). The text introduces the fat person to the doctor and explains her boundaries and requirements regarding her weight. Blog commenter Sticky did much the same thing in person:

> When I met with the new doctor for the first time, I immediately launched into a speech about how I don't need diet advice, need her to treat me beyond weight, blah blah. I ended it with asking if she felt she could treat me without focusing on my weight. She said yes, and that was that. I was very nervous and teary about it though. I even wrote a few things down to say.

On *Shapely Prose*, blog commenter JupiterPluvius has no problem with ending an appointment with an uncooperative health care provider, saying, "This appointment is over. I need to leave now." One fat acceptance member, Stef, maintains a fat friendly health care professional list (found at http://cat-and-dragon.com/stef/fat/ffp.html) that allows people to find doctors who will treat them without making an issue of their weight.

The nature of the Fatosphere as a digital community adds another element to resisting medical rhetoric, and is an example of the power of the Fatosphere for the individual—the social construction of knowledge online. In other words, together these fat individuals come to an understanding of what is true for them.

To combat the dominant rhetoric, bloggers often take common assumptions about fat or anything in the media dealing with fat—a research study, a newspaper article, an online posting, or an advertisement—and examine ideas and conclusions together with their readers. The members of the community examine the wording, the research methods, and the conclusions of articles looking for flaws, fallacies or legitimacy within them. They quickly point out any obvious or hidden fat prejudice within the pieces. Together, the community will come to an understanding of the relevance of data or the lack of legitimacy within the piece, slowly building an accepted core of knowledge that the community agrees upon.

An excellent example of this occurred when the Fatosphere closely examined a study of the Amish that concluded genetic predisposition to fat could be overcome by exercise. The authors of the study argued that genetically fat individuals could stay thin by participating in "about 3 to 4 hours of moderately intensive physical activity, such as brisk walking, house cleaning, or gardening." In a post on the blog *Fatistician,* Shinobi42 asserted that it is unrealistic to expect the average American to live like the Amish. In posts on their own blogs, bloggers Bronwen and April D both emphasized that expecting an individual to exercise three to four hours a day is not realistic. On the blog *A Day in the Fat Life,* Bronwen argued that such extreme measures were not feasible:

So, now, besides eating a starvation diet, I also have to

exercise for four hours a day? Ummmm, in what universe is that really a viable solution?

On a post entitled "Better Things I Could Do With the Time," April D provided a list of other things she could do with the time, including belly dancing and her homework. Bloggers also questioned how the results would be spun in the media. Blogger *Living 400 lbs* argued that the study is "not about weight loss," but that the media would portray it with that spin anyway. "Yeah, whatever you do," Shinobi42 said, "don't interpret this study to mean anything about how it might be unrealistic to expect every person on earth to be thin while living a modern lifestyle." Additionally, blogger Sandy Szwarc at *Junkfood Science* explains problems with the data itself:

> Despite the great import being given this study's findings as a prescription for weight management, a prudent precaution is to remember that it was an epidemiological data dredge study. Anytime we throw enough variables into a computer, it's bound to find some correlations, but that doesn't mean they mean anything. This study is no different.

Fat individuals have learned to gather fat-supportive facts and present them to doctors as an argument for good care. The community at *Big Fat Blog* put together a fact sheet called *Big Fat Facts*, on weight loss and fat health from a fat pride point of view.

Together, individuals in the Fatosphere are learning to reinterpret the dominant rhetoric in a more fat-friendly light.

Humor as Resistance

Humor has proven to be one of the strongest ways that fat individuals combat oppression, a strategy and experience that hooks does not discuss in her ideology of domination. We see humor employed as a strategy of resistance most especially in the Fatosphere.

Some members of fat acceptance are aware that they use humor to undermine the dominant rhetoric. For instance, the term "death fat" is proposed by Lesley Kinzel as an alternative to the medical term "morbidly obese." In "Death Fat Contextualized" Kinzel explains that "death fat" was supposed to be funny, a way to undermine medical terms with negative connotations. The blogger explains:

> Laughter relieves stress; for example, the stress of being a fat person who is routinely told—by an individual and/ or by cultural discourse as a whole—that you are morally suspect, intellectually-inferior, physically-disgusting, and/or ultimately doomed to die (unlike, uh, everyone else).

On the same post, JupiterPluvius enthusiastically responds that "death fat" is "subversive and sarcastic and delightful!" In the same discussion on "death fat," BrokenKali notes that humor helps "point out that it's not our bodies that are the problem, but attitudes."

The Fatosphere provides many of examples of fat individuals using humor to undermine the dominant rhetoric. Some terms are meant to undermine the belief that fat people have voracious appetites. The term "baby donuts" is perhaps the most prominent of these examples. "Baby donuts" first appeared in a conversation on *Shapely Prose* discussing an article written by Paul Campos addressing the ridiculousness of the term "overweight." The conversation that inspired the term went like this:

> **Stephanie:** Because, clearly, people with a BMI over 30 aren't human or anything. *grmph*...*goes to eat another sandwich, with processed cheese and white bread and OMG mayonnaise*

Kateharding: Well, personally, I eat babies, but that's just me. Not all fat people do.

Fillyjonk: Don't fill up on babies! Leave room for donuts.

Kateharding: Oh, never fear. I'm all about the baby-flavored donuts. With extra high-fructose corn syrup. And extra baby.

Spins: Kate, have you got any fresh babies. I only have baby jerky, but apparently that's too full of salt to be healthy for me.

Yellowhammer: Mmmm, extra baby.

Sniper: Also, what about fat vegetarians who don't get to chow down on nice, fresh baby? Are there any substitutes? Bofy? Tofinfant?

RHC: [O]k, the eating babies and donuts and baby flavored donuts was just too funny. Thank GOD for you guys. With gems like these, I can read those asinine comments on the Campos article and still laugh.

The phrase "baby donut" is often used as a sarcastic replacement for the meme of fat people sitting around eating donuts all day combined with the fear of fat people because they might eat your baby.

Another common phrase associated with the appetites of fat individuals is "two whole cakes," originated by blogger Lesley Kinzel. Kinzel explained exactly what the phrase meant to her:

To me, two whole cakes represents the absurd hyperbole associated with weight and body size. It acknowledges that there are folks out there, in numbers, who sincerely believe that all fatasses everywhere do things like sit down and eat two whole cakes on a regular basis, whence their fatness is maintained or improved upon. The over-the-topness of not one, but two whole cakes highlights the ridiculousness of beating myself up for choices that, ultimately, are not going to ruin my life or anyone else's.

Other terms are meant to underscore the fearmongering of the "obesity epidemic." The phrase "Booga Booga Booga obesity epidemic," coined by Meowser, is meant to undermine the fear induced by headlines claiming early death for fat individuals. Also, "teh obese," an homage to the misspellings of the LOL cats found at ICanHasCheezeburger.com, is meant to undermine the "Othering" factor of the commonly used term "the obese," a term Laurelhel argues is dehumanizing.

Finally, a more recent example taking place in the summer of 2012. In response to a commenter on the blog *Feministe* calling soda "an agent of obesity," Brian Stewart of *Red No. 3* started a whole movement of fat secret agents and super heroes. He portrayed himself as "Nick Fatty—Agent of Obesity," to which Kath Read, *Fat Heffalump*, became "The Incredible Bulk." Soon afterward more "agents" joined the fray: Enorma Sass, Zoe Cupcake, Big Libertine, Captain Fatalicious, and so on. Brian even created a seal and some superhero movie posters. He explains his response:

> They demand to have our bodies acknowledged as a grave threat to all of civilization. We respond by imagining a network of super spies with silly puns for codenames. Seems like an appropriate response to me.

Humor is a powerful way that fat individuals can fight the dominant rhetoric. Responses to fat hate help fat individuals deflect all of the negative messages sent toward them. These memes and movements show that humor also works to bond the fat community together.

Interestingly enough, hooks never mentions humor in her writing. However, my research suggests that it certainly seems effective as a strategy for undermining the dominant rhetoric.

Rhetoric & Conflicts within the Fat Studies Movement

Look, in the end, it comes down to a very old saying:
If you don't stand for something, you'll fall for anything.

We stand for fat positivity. For rejecting the constant barrage of societal messages telling us we're defective, worth less, hideous, deformed, and a plethora of other adjectives. We stand for taking care of your own health, whatever your personal definition of that is and without it being a relative meter stick for defining your worth as a human being. We stand for doctors treating us with dignity and care instead of with weight loss pamphlets and canned speeches. We stand for goddamn options when it comes to clothes, ffs.

We stand for something. And when we stop standing for it, the whole community falls. For anything.

Marianne Kirby

Like other social justice movements, conflict abounds within the fat acceptance movement—conflict that is often connected to words. As individuals fight the internalized belief system, they slowly move further and further from the standards of the status quo to belief systems that do not reflect the domination process. The process of moving away from such standards can create frustration and conflict both within the individual and within the community. Conflict is a natural part of the growth of the movement, which helps everyone negotiate the beliefs of the group as a whole.

As noted in Chapter 5: The Myth of Justified Oppression, because fat individuals can often lose weight for a time, there exists an added dimension to the experience of fat individuals in terms of oppression. However, we always see the desire for thinness as the desire to establish a position within the status quo.

In order to change this, hooks believes, current ideals of beauty and desirability must be critiqued while diversity should be embraced. The oppressed, hooks argues, must be aware that ideals of the dominant culture can permeate resistance movements in subtle ways. She also maintains that children are this system's "most vulnerable victims."

The dominant cultural ideals appear in conflict within the fat acceptance movement in many different conversations, but three areas are especially relevant: "in-betweenies" versus the "death fat," "good fatties" versus "bad fatties," and whether or not an individual can pursue weight loss and be part of the fat acceptance movement.

Levels of Fat

A repeated topic of conversation in the Fatosphere as well as in my focus group is the subject of levels of fat. A few ideas came out of this conversation: Is there such a thing as too fat, how fat is "fat," and the different experiences of individuals based on how just how fat they are. Death fat individuals feel that they are often considered too fat to be part of the movement. In a post on *Not a Pretty Girl*, Natalie explains how she views death fat and how she feels marginalized even within fat acceptance:

And that's one of the elephants in the room of fat acceptance. It's okay to be fat, but not too fat. If you're really fat, you'll be grudgingly accepted, but you'll be made aware of the fact that really, your body's not acceptable to them, either. If you're bigger than size 26 or heavier than 300 pounds, you're off in no-man's land. There's lip service paid to being accepting of all fat people, but I'm here to say that I'm not really feeling the love.

In the focus group, Vicky noted that though body acceptance has become more widespread, there appears to be a limit on acceptability. She sees it as, "Be fat, but not THAT fat." In a post on *The Rotund,* commenter Peggynature says that 300 pounds seems to be the magic number where acceptance stops:

> Something about that number, 300, carries really intense psychological weight with it. People really do believe that people are bed-ridden, or lifted out of houses on cranes, at 300 lbs (and that's not to denigrate people who do experience those realities—it's just that they tend to weigh closer to 1000 lbs. than 300). 300 seems to be the magic number at which acceptance of fat ENDS for most people.

Conversely, in-betweenies sometimes feel that they are not fat enough to be accepted into the fat acceptance movement. On *Not a Pretty Girl,* commenter Fat Brown Girl notes that at size 14 she feels "shunned for not being 'fat enough'. When I talked about my difficulties, it was like my problems didn't count until I weighed more." In the online focus group, Jessica mentioned feeling unwelcome in fat acceptance groups because she was not fat enough, a situation Julie had witnessed at fat acceptance events. In a post on *Shapely Prose,* Firefey and Individ-ewe-al talked about in-betweenies having "passing" privilege, which is being able to fit in with the accepted culture.

Yet in-betweenies can experience a particular type of pressure to lose weight, as blogger Nudemuse explains:

> One of the things that probably bothers me the most at this size is the assumption by the world at large that I am a work in progress. That I am at the midway point between some 'horrifying' before picture and the 'lovely' after picture. I think at the size I am which is probably a little larger than average in spots…it is [assumed] that I am actively losing weight.

So in-betweenies may be considered more acceptable, but have their own set of issues.

The conversation regarding levels of fat is repeated in the Fatosphere from time to time—for example, in September 2007 and again in May 2009. Most people who have been around any length of time appear to have negotiated this issue to a comfortable understanding, as illustrated by Kirby's post on "Smaller Fats and Larger Fats: Once More Round the Mulberry Bush." In this post, Kirby argues that smaller fat individuals belong in fat acceptance:

> A size 14 is considered fat by American society so a size 14 is fat. In other countries, the lines are drawn in different places. It does not lessen our experience, no matter what size we are, when a person who is culturally considered fat describes themself as fat.

Kirby argues that larger fat individuals often respond negatively to smaller fat individuals because "[w]hen a person who is not culturally defined as fat calls themself fat, it can be a totally anger-inducing thing because it lowers the bar for what fat IS, culturally speaking, and it is also an appropriation of labels." Yet, she notes, since women are taught to hate any extra weight, this will continue to happen. Kirby goes on to stress that the experience of a truly fat individual is different than that of an in-betweenie:

> There is a difference between not being able to find anything that fits you well and not even having the option of ill-fitting clothing period....Larger fats, meanwhile, get to worry about things like load capacity. The Wii Fit board is apparently only rated up to 300 pounds. That actively [bars] many larger fat people from playing with it. 300 pounds is the common limit to scales. 300 pounds is the common limit for people expecting you to be utterly bed-ridden.

Apparently, Kirby was responding to someone who claimed that acknowledging such differences creates a hierarchy within fat acceptance, a fact that Kirby argued against. Instead, she says that it is important to recognize the differences and respect them. Julia, on the same post, declares that "[listening] and acknowledging the diversity of experience helps us learn empathy and understanding. It strengthens us," while Lori explains that "there is a big difference between noting privilege (which I do think those of us who have more 'socially-acceptable' fat bodies have) and dismissing another person's lived experience."

The conflict between death fat individuals and in-betweenies does reflect the dominant belief that less-fat individuals are superior. On the whole, the community seems to agree that fat prejudice happens on a spectrum—different in different situations (for example, in Hollywood, people are fat at size 6)—and that we need to explore and acknowledge the issues at all aspects of that spectrum.

Good Fatty vs. Bad Fatty

Another area of conflict within the fat acceptance movement that reflects the dominant rhetoric is illustrated by participants in the Fatosphere often struggling with the idea of the "good fatty" vs. the "bad fatty." They often fight the stereotypical view of fat individuals, found in one study by Puhl and Brownell as "mean, stupid, ugly, unhappy, less competent, sloppy, lazy, socially isolated, and lacking in self-discipline, motivations, and personal control." In an attempt to combat these stereotypes, many fat individuals discuss their own healthy eating and exercise habits.

One of the reasons these individuals discuss such topics is that many have experiences of not being believed. For example, as discussed earlier, blog commenter Marshmallow conveyed that her doctor did not believe her when she described her eating and exercise habits. In the fat acceptance communities, fat individuals feel safe to discuss their healthy eating and exercise habits, knowing that in this arena they will be believed.

However, these discussions have created conflict in the Fatosphere and other fat acceptance realms—conflict which reflects the dominant rhetoric suggesting that health is an obligation of the person. In a society that assigns health a morally elevated value as much as the United States does, says Campos, fat individuals who practice healthy behaviors are more accepted than those who do not. Blogger Kate Harding points this out in a post entitled, "Good, Bad, Straw":

> In our efforts to find wider acceptance for fat people, it could be tempting to say, "Okay, well, they're ready to accept the 'good' fatties a little now, so the rest of you wait over there, and those of us with normal blood pressure and no eating disorders will come back for you later."

Harding goes on to argue that the good/bad fatty dichotomy is a "straw fatty" argument. These statements are relatively common in the Fatosphere, since the need to fight for the rights of all fat individuals, whether they are healthy or not, is a basic tenet of fat acceptance.

However, it is easier to sell the idea of a fat individual who is focused on healthy behaviors than one who is not. In the same post as Kate's comment above, Meowser talks about selling fat acceptance:

> But unfortunately, at this point in time, "But I DON'T stuff my face with donuts and I'm still fat" is a better opening shiv in the war against the haters than, "So WHAT if I stuff my face with donuts, is it any of your business?" Because people DO think it's their business.

By proving that individuals can be fat and fit, fat acceptance is more likely to gain ground.

When considering the feminist cause, hooks argues that "society is more responsive to those 'feminist' demands that are not threatening, that may even help maintain the status quo." Behaviors that are more in line with the status quo are more likely to be supported; therefore, "healthy" behaviors are more likely to be supported. Yet arguing that fat individuals deserve rights because a person can be fat and healthy can create an entirely different set of problems on the societal level, problems I explore in Chapter 17: Love in Action: Health At Every Size.

Once again, this situation presents a fat individual with an opportunity to step off the grid, to step out of the mindset of health as morality. As blogger Deeleigh says, "But the true rebellion is in making our own decisions and managing our own lives, not in living our lives as a reaction against healthism and the weight loss mentality." Blogger Lesley Kinzel explains that those who society labels as "morbidly obese" do not have to make up for their body size with healthy behavior:

> This here is a call to the morbid to out ourselves. You don't have to bike ten miles a day to make up for it. You don't have to be "healthy" by anyone's standards but your own. You don't even have to be totally 100% really for real in love with your body. You don't have to post pictures (unless you want to). You DO have to make an effort to not apologize. To not feel guilty (or ashamed). To just be yourself.

Subsequently, many individuals within the fat acceptance movement have chosen to fight for the rights of all fat individuals, not just the people who are trying to be healthy.

Dieting & the Fatosphere

Another conflict that appears in the Fatosphere is one that may be unique to fat oppression: Can individuals who choose to diet be part of the fat pride community? This conversation comes up repeatedly in the Fatosphere. In line with that question, can a person be a fat activist, yet try to lose weight?

The Fatosphere buzzed with regard to both of these questions after Hanne Blank, author of *Big, Big Love,* attempted to lose weight and blogged about it in September 2007 (a blog post that is no longer available). Harding and Kirby argued that dieting does not belong in the Fatosphere and that you cannot be a fat activist and diet. On the other hand, blogger Natalie at *Not a Pretty Girl* accuses fat acceptance members of moral judgment: "The party line is that if you do lose weight, you need to be apologetic about it and explain that it was accidental, that it just happened." Natalie makes an argument commonly heard in these conversations, which is that weight loss for health should be acceptable:

> I need to start taking better care of my body. And that means forcing myself to exercise (which I'm doing a terrible job at so far) and refraining from eating so much crappy food (limited success on that front). And you bet your damn bippy that if I manage to lose some weight... I'm going to be happy about it.

Kirby, writing as *The Rotund,* explains her thinking in a comment on Natalie's blog:

> [I]t is emphasized time and again that it isn't about making value judgments of people who choose to diet. It's about the way intentionally seeking to lose weight and promoting a fat accepting attitude have two very different goals. And no one, absolutely no one, has claimed that fat activists have never felt a desire to be thinner. In our society, that is pretty much completely unavoidable.

Natalie stopped blogging about fat after this interchange. Both Kirby and Harding argue that dieting should be avoided because it does not work, while the HAES approach has better success with improving health. Additionally, Harding asserts that "[d]eliberately trying to lose weight is, by definition, not accepting your own fat."

Another argument in support of prohibiting diet talk in the Fatosphere is so common that it has a Fat Hate Bingo square: "[Y]ou're endangering the rights of dieters!" Kirby emphasizes the idea of "unprivileging" dieting. That is, "[M]aking it not the default pursuit of women and men whose bodies differ from what is perceived as the social ideal."

Through the years, the general consensus in the Fatosphere appears to be "love the dieter, hate the diet." In other words, a person who is dieting is welcome in the communities as long as they do not talk about their diet or how much weight they have lost.

When the conversation appeared again in November 2008, Lindley at the blog *LivingXXL* explains that diet talk, not the dieter, is the problem:

> If you're dieting, I don't care. It's none of my business. But can you please take it elsewhere? The fat acceptance community is just not the place to discuss it. There are a billion other places on the web where you can talk about dieting....However. The rest of us need our own safe space, one that's free of diet talk.

Surprisingly, finding a safe space from diet talk is a great challenge to the Fatosphere. In response to Lindley's post, an anonymous commenter wrote, "You sound like you expect to be insulated from things because you don't like them." An anonymous commenter, known as A fat person, raged in response:

> Fat activists have no right to be free from your hatred and bigotry. How dare we try to find one small place of refuge in a world that is obsessed with talking about how we ought not be and about all the ways we should try not to be. How FUCKING rude of us to want to have our beliefs respected enough to not be repeatedly

subjected to discussions which belittle and marginalize us. How dare we try to carve out some little niche where we can go to not be bombarded with diet talk and calorie counting and "cheat days" which reduce our bodies to an objectionable other under a false veneer of "betterment". A betterment defined by attacking and insulting that which we are and that which we are overwhelming likely to continue to be no matter how many carbs get counted.

The need for a diet-talk-free zone is so important to many Fatosphere bloggers that somewhere, either on their main pages or in their comments policy, they announce that they are a diet-free or diet-talk-free zone. For instance, on the main page of the *Fatshionista* blog, Lesley Kinzel calls her blog "diet-free." Kirby calls her blog an "anti-dieting zone." Rachel at *The-F-Word* has a long list of unacceptable comments including: "Comments promoting weight-loss for the sake of weight-loss, commercial diets or other dieting behaviors" and "personal 'success' stories of how you lost weight, and we can too!" This argument in the Fatosphere shows how powerful the dominant rhetoric can be and how hard bloggers must fight to keep that rhetoric from their safe spaces.

In the past, I argued loudly and vehemently that dieters could not call themselves fat activists. I still think someone who is dieting undermines their beliefs when they try to balance fat activism and dieting. Yet I have come to understand that fat pride is a process, not an event, a situation that Australian researchers Marissa Dickins and colleagues found as well in their article "The role of the [F]atosphere in fat adults' responses to obesity stigma."

When fat individuals find fat acceptance and open their minds to the idea, they usually go through a time of cognitive dissonance, a time of split minds. They want to lose weight, yet think that fat individuals deserve respect and acceptance. And for a time they go back and forth between these two very divergent ideas. Most people, it seems, eventually give up dieting completely or leave fat acceptance completely.

One other common issue that rocks fat acceptance communities fairly regularly is white privilege and meeting the needs of people of color within the movement. I look at this issue in Chapter 18, "Fat Acceptance for Everyone."

What all of these conflicts come down to is a fear of being excluded—a feeling many fat individuals know well. Any hint that inclusion might be endangered brings out strong feelings in a person. Hence the conflicts in the Fatosphere.

CHAPTER 14
Hooks vs. Foucault: Power & Resistance

When examining hooks' idea of resistance, we see a major difference between her philosophy and the ideas of Foucault, often the theorist of choice when considering power relations. Foucault provided few solutions to the internalization of bio-power, what Foucault calls techniques for subjugating bodies. This situation is not surprising, since he views resistance as an inevitable part of the power structure and gives the individual very little agency to change the power dynamic. He sees resistance as a permanent part of the power dynamic that shifts the status quo but never moves beyond it—the grid of intelligibility: "[T]he moving substrate of force relations which, by virtue of their inequality, constantly engender states of power."

Foucault claims that the resistance-power interaction is a continuing dynamic that will never be resolved, just changed—a bit of a fatalistic viewpoint. Actually, Foucault's grid of intelligibility did show up in my research. As fat individuals learn to speak out and resist the dominant beliefs, they find that the dominant condition seeks yet again to establish supremacy. Whether it is having fat acceptance language co-opted or fat acceptance being seen as an excuse, fat individuals see that the dominant rhetoric finds ways to undermine resistance. We see Foucault's grid at work in this situation, yet hooks' ideas are also in evidence.

In hooks' view resistance leads to the destruction of the power structure, and the individual can be the source of change by focusing on self-recovery. Unlike Foucault's fatalistic point of view, hooks desired an end to the domination dynamic, providing a more utopian—perhaps a bit too utopian—solution to power relations.

These ideas of hooks' add to our understanding of resistance because she provides an alternative to theorists such as Foucault who see resistance as futile. She believes that resistance is healing, that sustained resistance provides strength and power, that it "can protect us from dehumanization and despair." In my research, participants started healing by resisting the oppressor within, and then healed even more by resisting external forces of oppression.

Resistance also normalizes the oppressed condition. In this case, it makes the abnormal body more acceptable. By having fat bodies be visible, whether in purposeful activist situations or just daily life, the fat body can be seen as a normal human variant rather than a deviant condition that must be corrected.

The road to fat liberation and consequent resistance for the individual is complicated and filled with emotions (anger, for instance), frustrations (conflicts within the FA movement, for example), and negotiations (whether or not to allow diet talk). However, by resisting, fat individuals are healing, becoming empowered, and believing that they deserve what all humans deserve—to be seen as more than just a deviant body. Consequently, hooks' idea of resistance as healing is exemplified by the Fatosphere and fat acceptance populations.

Though accepting the fat body seems like a never-ending battle, progress is being made. Technical communication professor Amy Koerber has commented that enough disruption of the cultural norms may cause the norms to change, a situation that fat activists continue to strive for. Rhetorician Krista Ratcliff exemplified the fat individual's experience of disrupting the norms:

> Even as a person invokes personal agency to interrupt unethical discourses or unethical cultural structures and practices, that person cannot control the effects of her or his interruption. Sometimes, the interruption is successful; sometimes, partial; sometimes, unsuccessful. Whether successful or not, interruptions have consequences.

At times, such as when resistance is seen as an excuse for staying fat or when receiving catcalls while choosing to be visible, the consequences can be painful for the fat individual.

Language, too, is one place this disruption becomes evident. Language can change things, hooks argues: "[L]language disrupts, refuses to be contained within boundaries." She asserts that by breaking the silence, by using the "liberatory voice," oppressed individuals find connection as well. Fat individuals have found that language can be a source of power, a survival mechanism in a fat-hating world.

CHAPTER 15
Knowledge & Resistance

Victimization is another issue that a fat individual must face. One way individuals in the Fatosphere avoid victimization is to come to an understanding of the fat condition outside of the kierarchy's system. We see an understanding of this when members of the Fatosphere deconstruct the dominant messages and reconstruct a shared knowledge in terms of fat acceptance.

When considering knowledge creation in online environments, the first thing to understand is that "knowledge is always situated," and since online experiences "disrupt the sense of bounded space," online environments become an important element in knowledge creation, according to rhetor Beatrice Smith. Laura Gurak claims that online discussions can "be used to focus and shape an alternative vision," a situation we see when bloggers in the Fatosphere deconstruct negative messages about fat and then reconstruct them in terms of fat acceptance. Online discourse also produces a disruption of societal ideals, or a location of resistance in the dominant messages, so that "online interaction can be politically meaningful," says Amy Koerber. So the nature of the online environment adds to the power of the Fatosphere as a source of resistance and a way to avoid victimization.

Group identity is an important factor in knowledge creation online. Authors of online texts attempt to appeal to the user's group identity as well as their own individual identities, says technical communication scholar Barbara Warnick. Group identity is an identity that users create as authors "not only of text, but of themselves, constructing new selves through social interaction," argues James Zappen, a professor of communications and media.

These group identities also work to constrain members of online communities. As Koerber noted, whether it be online or real life, "people are subject to multiple discursive constraints." The conflicts in the Fatosphere reflect these constraints in the ways the group constructs its identity and parameters together.

This chapter shows resistance working in the lives of fat individuals. Fat individuals are learning to resist the self-hatred of internalization; they are learning to resist the external dominant rhetoric; they are learning to use language and survival techniques to make this resistance possible. This resistance can be quite a challenge for the fat individual, as *Shapely Prose* commenter wriggles attests:

> I think fat acceptance is much harder than dieting, it is the road less travelled. It is condemned as ill-disciplined but I find it's not about that....It takes huge resolve to go against the establishment, the public and family and friends. Anyone who thinks you don't need discipline for that is an idiot.

Resistance to domination must be learned and then practiced, hooks argues. Fat individuals are practicing resistance in many different ways. These lessons are leading fat individuals to what hooks claims is the solution for domination—the incredible power of love, as we shall see in the next section.

Overcoming Oppression: The Power of Love

I realized, in that moment, that I have achieved something amazing. I have an incredible ability to love myself and to love how I look, for richer, for poorer, for thinner, for fatter, and til death do I part from this body. I can look in the mirror and love the woman I see no matter what size she is and no matter what society might think she should look like.

This ability to see myself with love goes beyond dresses and goal weights. I weigh more than I ever have, and I love myself more than I ever have. I've stripped away the conditions I previously attached to self-love, and it feels so good that I feel unstoppable.

Golda on *Body Love Wellness*

As Golda found, it is possible to love the fat body even in a fat-hating world. Given that American society's unsuccessful attempts at weight loss are not the solution to fat prejudice (changing the oppressed individual never is), members of the fat acceptance movement have put into action hooks' potential solution to oppression of all kinds—what she calls "love"— in order to overcome domination.

As noted in Chapter 1 and explained by Sonja K. Foss, Karen A. Foss and Robert Trapp, hooks' concept of love is not the sentimental feeling we usually associate with the term, but rather a force that fights against dehumanization. In hooks' conception of love, everyone is understood, appreciated and valued. "This vision of relationships," hooks said, "where everyone's needs are respected, where everyone has rights, where no one need fear subordination or abuse," is a vision that contradicts the dynamic of domination. The job of the resistors is to create "a critical discussion where love can be understood as a powerful force that challenges and resists domination," she says, arguing that love can lead to liberation for both the oppressed and the oppressor:

> The moment we choose to love we begin to move against domination, against oppression. The moment we choose to love we begin to move towards freedom, to act in ways that liberate ourselves and others. That action is the testimony of love as the practice of freedom.

In hooks' eyes, the concept of love is a solution to oppression. Her idea of love closely resembles Kenneth Burke's idea of identification. Burke argues that humans are by nature divided and that through communication can find a way to identify— that is, find a location of connection—with each other. Rhetor Krista Ratcliffe explains what this means in terms of listening, an important part of rhetoric:

> [U]nderstanding means listening to discourse not for intent but with intent—with the intent to understand not just the claims but the rhetorical negotiations of understanding as well.

Ratcliffe continues to argue that we can choose conscious identification—that is, we can knowingly choose to connect.

In my own experience, I see this as "love" the verb rather than "love" the feeling. That ooey-gooey feeling we usually associate with the term "love" is wonderful, but fleeting even in the best of relationships or situations. What is not fleeting is the choice to act lovingly, either toward ourselves or others. We always have the choice to connect, to see behind pain and anger and difference, to find commonality.

So what would hooks' vision of love, this choice to connect, look like in terms of fat pride? For the most part, the fat acceptance movement calls for all individuals—but most especially fat individuals—to accept their bodies while demanding that fat individuals be treated with respect and value. This love takes many forms, my research reveals: finding love for the fat body (one's own body and others' bodies) in and of itself, the acceptance and love for all bodies, choosing loving actions toward the body (the HAES philosophy), and creating a loving and accepting environment to discuss fat acceptance.

Love can improve health issues that weight-loss attempts cannot, while also providing a solution for issues of fat prejudice, including eliminating internalized fat hatred within fat individuals. By looking at the fat acceptance movement and the Fatosphere through hooks' concept of love, we see what it means to love a fat body in a fat-hating world.

In this section I will examine what it means to love the fat body, how the HAES approach is a form of love in action, how fat acceptance holds implications for everyone in American society, and how self-love and activism can interact.

CHAPTER 16
Loving the Fat Body

And I realised, the reason that I was able to see this young woman's beauty, despite the fact that she clearly didn't meet modern social standards of beauty, and despite the fact that she was dressed in a way that a year or so ago I would've thought was just "unnecessary" for someone with her body type, was that I've finally, finally stopped looking at fat people in a [judgmental] way.

Maddie on a post called "fat girl in tight clothes"

As the quote above attests, fat individuals have found that loving and/or accepting the fat body can be a place of empowerment and strength. Loving a body that is not touted as beautiful by the dominant rhetoric can be a powerful position for the oppressed, hook notes; seeing an unaccepted body as beautiful can be empowering.

We see this in discussions on the Fatosphere. When an online discussion of research showing that fat individuals can be healthy turned to the topic of anger at being fed the opposite belief, blog commenter KMTBERRY noted that loving all bodies can help with feelings of rage. Another commenter, Maddie, notes that as she accepted herself and found acceptance for other fat individuals: "[I]t seems that the internal has turned outwards, and now I can look at other fat people without judging them."

Self-love can be a "radical political agenda," hooks argues. In other words, self-love in the face of society's judgment can be an act of resistance.

Participants in the focus group also discussed what it meant to accept and love themselves and to be loved and accepted. Julie noted that members of the fat pride movement often have better body images than almost everyone else within our society, loving and accepting her body's "physicality, the actual and symbolic space it takes up, and the messages it conveys to others about my strength and power." Vicky spoke of being supported and surrounded by love at a NOLOSE conference, feeling proud of being fat. For these individuals, love has helped them come to accept their own fat bodies.

Amlys explains a brilliant idea that shows love in action. On *Dances with Fat,* she wrote:

> After poking around the SA blogosphere, I started challenging myself to find one beautiful thing about fat women. Even if it was, "I like her earrings." Eventually, I started seeing beautiful things about their bodies, too. It became an automatic response to fatness—looking for one beautiful thing. I don't see anything that upsets me—[I] don't associate adiposity with being unattractive anymore. Now, I instinctively look for one beautiful thing about every person I see, fat or thin. I truly have found myself to be accepting of all sizes—I don't see size anymore, just that one beautiful thing that I find about that particular person.

We can see that loving and accepting the fat body can be healing for fat individuals.

However, Marianne Kirby argues that the "love your body" meme can be problematic. Kirby explained her issues with the concept on her Tumblr page:

It's very much coming from a place where people want to feel good about themselves and to help other people feel good about themselves, too.

But it homogenizes bodily experience and feeling—basically it dictates the One True Way people are "supposed" to feel about their bodies. And that skeeves me. Because there are lots of reasons people have complicated relationships with their bodies—from trans identity to disability to body dysmorphia in general and so on.

I also think that for someone just coming off a diet or an eating disorder, loving the body is far too tall an order.

Blogger Nudemuse had another take on the idea of loving the fat body. She argues that like any relationship, love for the body can be difficult:

> Love as a thing as a changing breathing difficult thing is never perfect and smooth and wonderful. Not our relationships with our friends, not with our families, not with anything or anyone not ever.

> What I don't understand is how so many people conflate this perfect love scenario when we talk about our bodies. Or that to love this thing, our bodies means that we won't ever have an issue with them....

> I am for [l]oving your body enough to understand that sometimes it's going to fail. Sometimes your body is going to be fucked.

> Just like in any relationship, you're going to fight. Sometimes it's going to be ugly and really fucking hard. Sometimes, loving your body means accepting that no, you won't walk normally or that no, you won't be thinner or no, your skin won't ever be perfect.

I agree with this idea of a relationship with the body and all that it implies—complication, mixed feelings, and the like. I found loving my body to be unfathomable at first, and something I could not force. Feeling love for the body can be incredibly challenging, and really is unnecessary, in my experience. However, I found that *accepting* my body is absolutely vital. The ideas expressed in the Serenity Prayer, popular in recovery circles, are applicable in this situation:

> Grant me the serenity to accept the things I cannot change, to change the things I can, and the wisdom to know the difference.

I spent many years hating my body and not accepting it for what it was. I did myself a great deal of emotional and physical damage with that state of mind. For that reason, I had to make acceptance important. I could change some things, such as becoming stronger and more flexible. However, after thirty years of trying to lose weight, I had to accept my weight as it was.

I also must accept my body as it is before I can make any improvements. I have to accept my current level of fitness before I can make progress, or I wind up injured and in worse shape. I have to accept my health as it is before I try to improve it.

To me, feeling love for the body is not as important as accepting it and honoring it. Yet I think that acceptance and honor are forms of love—the kind of love hooks talks about, love in action. I can always choose to act lovingly toward my body, no matter how I feel about it. I can always choose to connect with my body. I can always choose to feed and exercise it according to its needs. I cannot control how I feel about it.

So in my viewpoint, trying to feel love for my body really is not important. Choosing to treat my body with respect and honor, to act lovingly toward it, is vital.

Looking at these different viewpoints on loving the body demonstrates that the idea is not a straight-forward, well-defined concept. Loving the body is situational and individual, and its meaning and relevance must be discovered for each person.

Yet the actual experience of discovering love and acceptance for our bodies can be a liberating experience for the fat individual. Blogger April D explains how she found acceptance by letting go of limitations in terms of acceptance:

> So many of us attach limitations or "only when" conditions to self-acceptance!! For me it has been a variety of things from particular weights, fitting into a certain piece of clothing, getting a specific grade...and you know, even if/when I DID reach whatever limiting condition I'd put on my own self-love and happiness...I'd change the rules on myself and make up a whole NEW set of even more narrowly restrictive conditions...

> Huzzah for getting to the "unstoppable" feelings finally and putting aside that feeling that there is always some other limit, just out of reach, beyond which true happiness lies!

Some fat individuals used to think self-acceptance would come with weight loss, though many individuals have chosen to accept themselves as they are today. Blog commenter Peggynature argues that "[t]he promise of self-acceptance is not the same as the promise of a new diet," stating that the diet promises sweeping life changes that prove to be unrealistic. On the other hand, self-acceptance provides true change, but at a slower pace. In a post on *The Rotund,* commenter Twistie asserts that accepting the body as is instead of needing it to change is a huge mental health boost.

Some people found that self-acceptance and self-worth are not a constant—rather, they require continual work to maintain. In the same post on *The Rotund,* commenter Caseyatthebat explains her process for reaching self-acceptance:

> I find more self-acceptance at the higher range, which leads to better self-care, which (for me) leads to the lower

range, which…you get the picture. Maybe genuine self-acceptance is like walking on solid ground after being on choppy seas, and it requires some time before one fully gets one's land legs.

Blogger and commenter Wellroundedtype2 says that she found detachment regarding her weight to be her goal, since "my weight goes up sometimes, it goes down sometimes, but what I can control is how kindly I treat myself about it."

That self-acceptance also provides fat individuals with compassion for others who are still in the struggle to care for themselves. As one blog commenter, AW, said, "I can empathize with anyone, of any size, who projects society's hate onto herself."

Self-acceptance can lead fat individuals to happier, more contented lives.

Knowing the Self

Learning to love the self can take many forms, including the ability to know oneself. Domination destroys individuals' ability to know their own selves, hooks asserts; as individuals recover from this violation, they find that internal being yet again, seeing themselves as more than just "the condition of domination."

Participants in the focus group spoke of the experience of having their entire being defined by being fat and having to redefine themselves when the dominating condition is taken away. Both Vicky and Nicole experienced this condition of defining themselves as other than fat when interacting with individuals in an advocacy group. Nicole spoke of perceiving herself as just a person, rather than a fat person, for the first time while playing Pictionary at a NAAFA event. Vicky talked of having to look at herself as a person rather than a fat person:

[T]he No[L]ose conference was the first time I ever spent concentrated time in the presence of so many fat people who were not trying to lose weight—or weren't discussing it anyway even if they were. There was so much power and acceptance there. Being among all these fat people forced me to look at who I was as a person as opposed to who I was as a fat person. The primary way I identified myself in the world was, all of a sudden, in this group, not the primary way I was identified.

This shift from being a fat person to just a person transforms the way fat individuals see themselves and their places in the world.

Relationships

Being loved for who they are has helped many fat individuals find self-love as well. In the focus group Nicole, Melissa and Susan all mentioned that being loved by a partner helped them come to love and accept themselves even more. In a discussion looking at self-loathing on the blog *Shapely Prose,* commenter estrella notes the power of being loved for herself, both to her own feelings about herself and her ideas of what attraction means:

> In recent years I've been with someone who—for the first time ever—makes me feel downright sexy. He loves my body and takes every chance to tell me. He's slim and muscular (and prone to occasional dieting) but always makes me feel hot. This has done wonders (WONDERS!) for my body image—not because it's important what other people think, but because I've actually started to realize how subjective real attraction is, that the standards of beauty plastered all over the media are not necessarily what everyone truly finds attractive.

Blog commenter Emily notes in a conversation on *The Rotund* that being loved by her partner helped her love herself more and take better care of herself. So being loved and accepted by others can help a person love and accept themselves.

Yet not worrying about what others think can also be a form of self-love. As Jane wrote on a post called "The State of Independence":

> My self-worth is not determined by the size of my ass, the span of my belly, the jiggleliciousness of my upper arms, my stretch marks, or how this might determine how attractive or unattractive I am to others.

At times, not caring about what others think can also be a form of self-love.

Loving Children

Love and acceptance are particularly important for the children in our society—all children in our society, whether fat or not. When discussing the supposed "obesity epidemic," a common response is often, "Won't someone please think of the children?" This response is so common, in fact, that it has its own Fat Hate Bingo square. Fat children are, perhaps, the greatest casualties in America's war against fat (see Chapter 6: Is It Prejudice? for the discrimination and issues fat children face). Along with loving their own bodies, fat individuals have found that they need to act as advocates for fat children, teaching all children to love their own and others' bodies.

In a discussion concerning fat children on *Shapely Prose*, Summer says that parents must speak up for their children: "I do feel we have to be vocal advocates for our children and take on the powers that be." In the same post, withoutscene argues, "I think one of the best things you can do as a parent is to NOT DIET or obsess about weight." Heather goes on to say that she does not allow her daughters to talk about the weight of others or others to talk about her daughters' weight. "There is plenty of time for the world to teach them to hate themselves," she explains, "my daughter is NOT going to be poisoned if I can help her." Continuing the discussion, commenter fashionablenerd describes her way of handling a child's bad day:

> This is what parents who have fat kids can do: keep telling their kids that no matter what, their worth isn't measured by pounds. Even if you think it's not [going to] stick (especially when they have a REALLY bad day and come home in tears), they'll remember that there was someone in their lives that accepted them. And that self esteem and acceptance is the best gift you can give to anyone.

The love and advocacy of children who are struggling with body image is supported by hooks' ideals. When speaking of the family, hooks argues that love should be the central guiding principle. By focusing on combating the negative images of the dominant rhetoric and supporting the self-esteem of children, individuals can show love for their children and show their children how to love themselves.

Acting lovingly toward the fat body is an important experience to fat individuals practicing fat acceptance. By choosing to love the fat body, fat individuals find a source of empowerment and liberation. Additionally, they learn to know themselves beyond just being a fat individual—they learn to know themselves outside of domination. Even advocating for fat children can be a form of loving the fat body for the fat individual.

Discussions in the Fatosphere and fat acceptance often show the HAES philosophy exemplifying that love for the fat body, as we shall see in the next section.

CHAPTER 17
Love in Action: Health At Every Size

And HAES is a practice based on working with your body where it is, and trying to improve your health regardless of whether it results in weight loss. It's not a state of being. This means people who weigh 600 lbs., people with disabilities, etc., can certainly practice HAES, though both the specific measures they take and the ultimate result may not be the same as those of someone smaller and/or who doesn't have disabilities.

Marianne Kirby

As the quote from Kirby exemplifies, the HAES philosophy is a practice, a practice in loving the self. Brazilian educator and critical theorist Paulo Freire argued that a solution to domination "cannot be achieved in idealist terms," but rather must be seen as a situation that can be transformed through action. The HAES philosophy is, in fact, a loving action on the part of the individual. Fat individuals take action and practice hooks' idea of love when they treat their own bodies lovingly and respectfully.

In this section I will look at how the HAES viewpoint affects the experience of fat individuals, as well as some of the struggles fat acceptance and the Fatosphere have experienced around the HAES philosophy, keeping in mind how the HAES ideas interact with hooks' idea of love. This philosophy is proving to be a powerful tool of both self-love and self-acceptance inside and outside of the fat acceptance movement.

To start with, members of the Fatosphere and the fat acceptance movement struggle to understand exactly what the HAES philosophy comprises. Of course, there is the definition provided by Linda Bacon that appears to be the overall accepted point of view:

- Accepting and respecting the natural diversity of body sizes and shapes.

- Eating in a flexible manner that values pleasure and honors internal cues of hunger, satiety, and appetite.

- Finding the joy in moving one's body and becoming more physically vital.

For another view, posting on *The F-Word,* guest blogger and nutritionist Deborah Kauffmann explained her definition of the HAES philosophy:

HAES is an approach to health and healthcare that promotes acceptance of natural body weight and an understanding that people come in all shapes and sizes. The HAES approach supports pleasurable and healthful eating that is based on internal cues of hunger and fullness as well as joyful movement.

But what exactly does this mean to a fat person's daily living? Blogger Fillyjonk explained how she sees the HAES perspective:

Anyone who's read [F]atosphere blogs for any length of

time will tell you that we are huge proponents of nutritious eating and regular movement, though for their own sake rather than for weight loss. Even the people who aren't all-HAES-all-the-time are interested in encouraging people to normalize their relationship with food—to stop seeing it as a source of sin or fear or love or comfort, not to turn around and make gluttony the main focus of our lives.

Fillyjonk also emphasizes that the HAES approach means "to care about your health MORE than you care about your weight, to care about your health independent of caring about your weight," which "takes vigilance." Kauffman states that practicing the HAES philosophy "just means taking care of ourselves without focusing on weight loss," which appears to be the overall attitude toward this concept in the Fatosphere and fat acceptance movement as a whole.

Fat individuals who practice the HAES approach often feel healthier, and can be healthier as determined by the dominant rhetoric, than those who diet. The HAES practice has a longer term positive outcome on health than dieting, improving health indicators (blood sugar, blood pressure, heart rate, cholesterol) for a longer period of time, Bacon has found.

When Kate Harding attacked diets presented under other names such as "lifestyle change" and "a whole new way of eating," saying that these changes did not lead to weight loss, Louise felt like Harding took away her hope of permanent weight loss, as exemplified by the following comment:

> I've been putting the hard work into changing my habits for two years, slowly getting healthier, [losing] weight, and being thrilled by the benefits. Your post depresses me horribly. I rather wish I hadn't found your blog.

Responses to this comment help clarify that feeling good is an emphasis of the HAES philosophy. Blogger Sweetmachine, who wrote on *Shapely Prose,* responded by highlighting that feeling good is enough of a reward for eating better, while filly-jonk explained that success in HAES philosophy terms is more consistent than dieting:

> Plus, that way you actually get to appreciate your healthiness and good feelings. If you're too focused on weight loss, on days when the scale goes up you feel crappy—even if you should be feeling nourished by your healthy foods and energized by your workouts. If you stop measuring your success and self-worth by numbers, you get to enjoy your real successes a lot more.

Fat individuals have found that by focusing on how they feel rather than on weight loss, they reach a sense of accomplishment.

Members of the fat acceptance movement and the Fatosphere often struggle with the differences, or lack of differences, between the HAES philosophy and dieting. This dilemma came out in a conversation regarding the ineffectiveness of diets. In a post on *Shapely Prose*, commenter Entangled, in discussing her exercise habits, made the following comment:

> I lost a significant (though in reality not that large) amount of weight over the past two years. Mostly because I decided I was going to teach myself to run. I didn't really change my eating habits (beyond stopping when full, not stuffed), but I got SERIOUSLY, DEPRESSINGLY, OBSESSIVELY anal about them.

> On the days on which I concentrate on my habits—the fact that I can now run five miles, that I finished my first 5K in under 32 minutes, that my intense intervals are upwards of 7.5 mph—I feel great. When I concentrate on the visual results of those efforts, I feel like crap. Terrified that things will change, depressed that it matters, obsessive about food again.

She thought her comment might be "teetering towards diet-talk." Blogger Harding responded positively, explaining how she saw diet-talk:

> [T]he diet talk I prohibit is the "Just do X and you'll
> lose the weight, and you'll feel better because you LOST
> WEIGHT!" Your comment, as I see it, was Health at
> Every Size talk. :)

This difference between HAES-talk and diet-talk reflects
another discussion that pops up on the Fatosphere—the fact
that some individuals will lose weight when practicing the
HAES approach. Commenter Caseyatthebat explains that she
experienced "some weird internal reverse-size acceptance" because of losing weight:

> I tell myself that I will eat healthfully, move my body in
> a joyful way and accept the result, but in my head the
> "result" should be no weight loss, and I'm having a hard
> time accepting that, for me, it might mean some weight
> loss.

When discussing the fantasy of being thin, commenter Mizerychik explained that she was one of the five percent who lost
weight and kept it off for more than five years, which made her
feel like she did not belong in the Fatosphere or fat acceptance
communities:

> I'm one of the 5%, and since reading more and more of
> the body acceptance movement, I kind of hate myself for
> it. Sometimes I feel like a traitor for reading this blog or
> that I don't belong, like I shouldn't comment because I
> am that freak of nature that often gets mentioned.

Members of the Fatosphere responded by emphasizing acceptance. Commenter Phledge responded by saying, "[D]on't
feel bad about that," emphasizing that mizerychik's body was
meant to be that way, while Meowser took the opportunity to
expand on the philosophy behind the HAES concept:

> "Anti-dieting" does not equal "stay fat at all costs so you'll

fit in with the rest of us fatasses." You, mizerychik, are a perfect illustration of what I'm talking about when I say, if you're truly meant to be a lot smaller than you are (or were), there's nothing I or anyone else can possibly do to stop you.

In her interview, Mustardseed put it succinctly when she explained that the HAES philosophy includes "accepting healthy thinness as well if that's what comes naturally." The differences between the HAES approach and dieting can be confusing, because many of the tenets appear to be the same; however, as these conversations and comments show, motivation tends to be the difference behind them. Additionally, weight loss diets follow rules, whereas the HAES philosophy encourages connection with and listening to the body.

Another place that controversy around the HAES philosophy comes into account is when dealing with eating disorders. Deborah Kauffmann explains that the HAES approach can be beneficial for someone with compulsive overeating or binge eating disorder, if they have help from a HAES nutritionist:

> It is extremely important for someone struggling with binge eating or compulsive eating to seek out a HAES nutritionist since dieting is one of the major causes of this type of disordered eating. Nutrition treatment for compulsive eating should involve assisting the client in eating enough total food according to internal cues of hunger and fullness, balancing the major nutrients (protein, fat, carbohydrate), including all liked foods, and eating mindfully to obtain the most pleasure from meals. It should also include HAES education regarding nutrition, the problems with dieting, principles of weight management and the relationship between weight and health.

Blog commenter Mshell67 came to *Shapely Prose* trying to figure out how a binge eater fit into fat acceptance:

I'm feeling awful right now because I feel conflicted about my eating. I definitely have an eating disorder (I woke up at 3:00 am and ate frosting out of the can) and other such shit. So yesterday I felt like crap about myself and ate myself into a binge-o-rama. So, my question is, would it be awful if I went to a counselor to discuss my binge eating issues in order to tame them a bit? What happens if I happen to lose weight? Am I a failure as a fat activist? Where do I fit in in this framework? Discuss please!! :)

In response, Kirby, writing as *The Rotund,* argued that mshell67 should go see a counselor and that suffering from an eating disorder and being a fat activist was not mutually exclusive. "Breaking away from disordered eating," she said, "is not the same as controlling and limiting your diet for the express purpose of losing weight." Fillyjonk noted that fat acceptance should support people with eating disorders:

I think you should expect—nay, demand!—that the fat acceptance movement buoy you up in your mission to eat in a way that is not harmful to you. Honestly, the fight against diets and the fight against binge eating or compulsive eating are two sides of the same coin: both are about healing our relationship with food, which is so drastically fucked up so early in life, and both are served by embracing HAES and unhitching health from weight.

Btsu believes that counseling would be a great idea, as long as it is a fat-neutral environment.

Considering these conversations, members of the Fatosphere view the HAES approach as a possible solution to eating disorders.

From the outside, the HAES concept can be seen as a form of hedonism. Blogger fillyjonk explains her experience with common responses to this philosophy:

But we're constantly being reviled—or at least treated with suspicion—for pimping overindulgence and inactivity. Why? Because we advocate treating yourself well, and that gets people's Puritan hackles up. Treating yourself well—doesn't that mean engaging in constant sinnery? Things that are good for you are supposed to feel like constant punishment, so if you're not punishing yourself, how can you ever do yourself good?

Yet the HAES philosophy is a solution that many members of the Fatosphere and fat acceptance have found to heal their past unhealthy relationships with food and their bodies. The HAES approach is an action that shows both love for the body and love for the self. Though some controversy appears in the Fatosphere over exactly what this philosophy means in daily life, how it is different from dieting, and how individuals with eating disorders deal with it, the HAES approach appears to be working for many members of the Fatosphere and fat acceptance communities. However, this philosophy brings with it some pitfalls for fat liberation, as will be discussed in the following section.

Rights for the Unhealthy

[T]he reality is that society is much more willing to accept a fat person who exercises than one who doesn't—and more willing still to accept a person who's trying to lose weight. In our efforts to find wider acceptance for fat people, it could be tempting to say, "Okay, well, they're ready to accept the 'good' fatties a little now, so the rest of you wait over there, and those of us with normal blood pressure and no eating disorders will come back for you later." Anyone who's worked in any social justice movement is familiar with that pitfall and why it must be avoided. Those who hew most closely to the dominant group's values (and/or appearance) are always the first candidates for "acceptability"—but taking that offer of acceptance while selling out those who are further away from the dominant group only reinforces the very values you're trying to dismantle. That's social justice 101.

Kate Harding in "Good, Bad, Straw"

Though the HAES philosophy is often the loving solution for the individual, fat activists warn that this area can be dangerous territory. If fat individuals are only allowed civil rights when they choose "healthy behaviors"—behaviors that may be defined as healthy by outside forces and may not have the fat individual's best interests at heart—a whole new slew of problems exist. On the *SFweekly* blog, Marilyn Wann said:

> As a fat activist, I often want to say, "But I'm healthy! Look, I eat my veggies and exercise." While it's fun to flout stereotypes, social justice is unacceptably precarious if it depends on good behavior, or on access to other flavors of unearned privilege.

Considering the context of this idea, though the dominant rhetoric still says that fat is undesirable and unhealthy and must be eliminated, even the media has started to put forth the idea that the HAES solution just might be possible or even ideal. A number of news outlets, including the *New York Times* and the *Los Angeles Times,* have run articles considering the HAES approach, or at least how fat individuals could be healthy without attempting to lose weight.

It appears that society is more willing to consider the idea that fat individuals deserve rights as long as the fat individuals are attempting to be healthy by society's standards. Yet a number of problems exist with this reasoning. The first problem is that if individuals should only deserve rights when they are attempting to be healthy, how do you tell? Do fat individuals have to wear monitors that prove they eat healthy foods (and, of course, you must define what "healthy foods" actually are) and exercise regularly? If the only fat individuals who deserve rights are those trying to be healthy, then what about the slender people who don't exercise and eat junk food?

This reasoning steps into a great quagmire of Big-Brother-type surveillance that has many potential pitfalls. Additionally, it immediately leaves out individuals who may be fat *because* of a health problem rather than the other way around. If an individual became fat because of an accident or disease, would they deserve rights? They are not healthy, yet that is no fault of their own.

These attitudes also present the danger of creating yet another prejudice—healthism, explained in Chapter 7: Comparing Prejudices and the Dynamics of Prejudice. If we allow healthism to take the place of fat prejudice, we once again create the same dynamic, the same ideology of domination, that hooks argues against. This also can take the fat individual into the good fatty/bad fatty debate explained in Chapter 13: The Power of Rhetoric.

Fat acceptance cannot be based on behavior, or we will continue to perpetuate domination.

CHAPTER 18
Fat Acceptance for Everyone

The fact is, fat activism is good for everybody, even people who are not fat, even people who don't know it exists or who don't think they need it. It's good for everybody to hear about fat activism, even in circumstances and scenarios when they weren't expecting to get hit with a dose of body love and social justice. Because everyone's got a body story; everyone's got an issue or an injury or a sad point or a sore spot. Fat activism starts with fat people but extends to everyone who lives in a culture in which beauty standards are dictated by a fatphobic culture; even folks who aren't fat have to live with the fear of getting fat, which is a powerful thing.

Lesley Kinzel on *Outfitblogging*

"[T]o be either dominated or dominating is a point of connection or commonality," providing a common ground for ending domination, hooks claims. She exemplifies this type of interaction by claiming that both the dominator and dominated will gain from the ending of oppression, and that this transformation must take place in both groups. The power behind domination, hooks notes, is fear, a term she describes as the following:

T]he primary force upholding structures of domination. It promotes the desire for separation, the desire not to be known. When we are taught that safety lies always with sameness, then difference of any kind will appear as a threat. When we choose to love we choose to move against fear—against alienation and separation.

When it comes to fat acceptance, everyone can benefit because everyone suffers from fat prejudice. As a society, we tend to think of fat issues in terms of white middle and upper class women. But the reality is that fat prejudice affects everyone. And while fat, white women make up the majority of the fat acceptance movement at this time, there is room, and need, for everyone who wants to further the cause of fat acceptance.

Non-fat People

When examining fat and the dominant culture of the United States, the connection between fat individuals and others takes on a particular relevance. As I discussed at length in the book *Talking Fat,* because of the belief that anyone can become fat, the fear of fat pervades our dominant culture. Additionally, the continual quest for the perfect body affects many people, particularly women, if we consider the context.

American women have practically made hating their bodies a pastime. According to the American Society of Plastic Surgeons, cosmetic surgery is up 69 percent since 2000. Women bond through talking about diets and denigrating their bodies, Hirschman and Munter report. Wann notes that "every person who lives in a fat-hating culture inevitably absorbs anti-fat beliefs, assumptions, and stereotypes, and also inevitably comes to occupy a position in relation to power arrangements that are based on weight." That being the case, when fat individuals fight to accept themselves as they are when considered very socially unacceptable, they provide an excellent example of body acceptance to those who may struggle with body issues at a smaller size.

In response to body denigration, slender people could be considered the enemy. For instance, American actress and comedienne Mo'Nique wrote a book entitled *Skinny Women are Evil*, in which she argues that skinny women are to be fought. However, non-fat individuals are also harmed by fat hatred.

Fat activists repeatedly argue against viewing skinny individuals as the enemy, claiming that thin bashing is part of fat hatred. In a conversation on privilege, blog commenter Kitty notes that "even 'backlash' against thin women is based in fat hatred because it comes from resentment at the thin-bashing person's 'failure' to be as close to the thin ideal as the person they're bashing." In the same post, pyewacket expanded upon this idea and explained her thoughts on how thin bashing was an element of fat hatred:

My own (former, I hope) backlash against thin women was based in fat hatred. I think it worked something like,

1. [P]eople hate my fat and assume I'm functionally and morally a slug.

2. I feel some vague sense of burning injustice about this.

3. Thin women are held up as the paragon of what I will never be. Ergo, jealousy.

4. The narrow line of acceptably thin is crossed and some chick starts showing rib-bones, which I KNOW is unhealthy because I've Read Articles Saying So, and yet she is still considered hotter than I am by leaps and bounds.

5. I sneer at this sellout Tool of the Establishment who is sacrificing her health for vanity (and oh God, the irony now).

6. The sneering spills over onto other thin people with less skeletal definition, because assumed moral superiority is like scratching the itch caused by the burning injustice in step 2.

Blogger fillyjonk explained the *Shapely Prose* viewpoint on thin women by admonishing a commenter, saying that "we don't insult or demean anyone's bodies here." She went on to explain that negative descriptions directed at thin women, such as calling them "sticks" or "boys," was not acceptable on that site. *The Rotund*, Marianne Kirby, summed it up nicely in a post entitled "Thank you, thin person."

The truth is that thin people have just as many body issues as fat people. They don't have them, necessarily, on a culture-wide level that leaves them struggling against ingrained body hatred to the degree that fat people do. But they do, as individuals who are products of the same world we fat people live in, have body issues.

Such a simple stance as seeing the perceived superior individuals as the enemy encourages individuals to ignore other forms of dominance and the role that individual plays in domination, hooks believes. For instance, when speaking of feminism, she notes that seeing men as the enemy is simplistic. Also, by doing so women do not "examine systems of domination and our role in their maintenance and perpetuation." She emphasizes that the idea is to move beyond contention to connection, where "dehumanization that characterizes human interaction can be replaced with feelings of intimacy, mutuality, and camaraderie." Again, hooks' ideas resemble Burke's identification, which, according to Krista Ratcliffe's feminist interpretation, "demands that differences be bridged."

This goal of connection is seen in the Fatosphere as well. Blog commenter Ailbhe illustrates this beautifully when she talks of being harassed for being thin:

I came here in tears one day because someone told me at the pool that they hated me for being thin, and I knew that *only in FA circles* was I guaranteed people who understood it wasn't a compliment and that I truly have no reason at all to even slightly associate my being thin with health.

Blogger and commenter Vesta44 explains that she would like "all bodies to be accepted as-is," and it is no better or fairer for thin individuals to be accepted based solely on how they look.

In a post on *Shapely Prose* discussing thin privilege, Morag wanted to know why thin individuals would frequent a fat acceptance site. The answers ranged across a spectrum of reasons: fighting the beauty myth and diet culture, dealing with eating disorders, handling fat family members, and helping other women—especially daughters—in loving themselves. For instance, LadyGrey frequented the site because she wanted to get beyond her judgment of fat people, while Ailbhe explained that she came mainly for her daughters:

I'm thin, but in my family of five sisters I am The Fat One (me and my 26-inch waist, I kid you not), and my daughters are similarly differently sized, and I want to know...how to make sure I don't fuck up any more than I have to. Clearly the world is very fucked up when sick, underweight girls are told they are either lucky or still too fat. Or both, sometimes.

If we can save the world while we're here, that's good too[.]

However, the overwhelming reason thin people read fat acceptance blogs tends to be self-acceptance and learning to appreciate their own bodies. Commenter Marste explained that she frequents *Shapely Prose* to "be reminded that my body size does not define my worth." Lis said that she identified "really strongly, with the sense that my body was always 'wrong', no matter what size I was." In terms of the dynamic surrounding fat prejudice, this would mean body acceptance for all, no matter their size.

Body dissatisfaction of thin or normal weight individuals can be a potentially dangerous area, however. The fact that non-fat people experience body dissatisfaction as well can be used to undermine the experience of the fat individual. This topic has been discussed a number of times in the Fatosphere, but was put into perspective by Kirby when she noted that:

> When a person who is not culturally defined as fat calls themself fat, it can be a totally anger-inducing thing because it lowers the bar for what fat IS, culturally speaking, and it is also an appropriation of labels. But because women especially are led to believe that ANY spare flesh (including, you know, the body fat required to keep people alive) makes them fat, we're going to keep running into this.

A common response to a fat individual speaking up about fat prejudice is the tendency to hear something along the lines of, "[B]ut thin women have body image issues as well," in a way co-opting and undermining the experience of the fat individual. Guest blogger volcanista tries to explain this tendency for skinny people to think they understand the fat experience:

> So, do some thin people get shit for being thin? Of course! People's bodies—especially women's bodies—are treated like public property all the time. And standing out in any way, especially in a physical way, often just seems to invite additional ridicule and mistreatment. Maybe that's why some thin people posit that they are the same, the fat experience and the thin experience. Getting teased and bullied for the shape and even the existence of your body, something you fundamentally can't change, and in many cases (for both the thin and the fat) something you

might try to change about yourself in hopeless and self-damaging ways—well, that shit hurts, and it's a deeply personal, formative experience. So I think that for some thin people, there's resentment when they hear a fat person complaining, like the fat person is trying to invalidate or one-up their own painful, skinny past. For others, there can be this pull to try to identify with the painful experiences of a fat person: to think you understand, to find a comrade who was also pushed around by the kids on the playground.

Though body image issues are a concern for most women in the United States, the fat experience also includes oppression. Fat acceptance is for thin people as well, but it is important not to allow that fact to undermine discussions on thin privilege and fat oppression.

Overall, fat acceptance and the Fatosphere encourage the participation of thin individuals. You will often hear thin individuals called "allies," but Marilyn Wann has argued against using this term on Facebook: "[W]eight-based oppression affects people of all sizes. I have always argued against calling thin people allies for this reason and also because I want to erase the imaginary (and shifting) line between 'fat' and 'thin,' not redraw and defend it."

However, fat individuals may struggle with accepting thinner individuals in fat acceptance spaces. Jo Geek explained these issues, as well as how a thin person might support fat acceptance, in a series of blog posts. Jo has condensed those posts into the following information, which she has given permission to include here.

How to Support Fat Acceptance as a Thin Person

BY JO CONKLIN
A.K.A JO GEEK

As a freshly minted fat activist in 2006, I struggled with the idea that I had spent my entire life fighting desperately and futilely towards being someone else's ideal, engaging in plenty of self-loathing and harm along the way. I had just had this massive paradigm shift with the realization that not only was I okay, but I had always been okay, even when everyone was telling me I wasn't. This was an amazing, liberating, and uplifting revelation. But it also made me angry. Really angry. I had wasted decades of my life hating myself unnecessarily and envying the effortlessly skinny girls who had everything I thought I wanted.

Fat acceptance activists don't become activists in a vacuum. We have to sort through, cope with, and fight against years of internalized messages. We have wounds. You are coming into a movement against a world where you are Marcia Brady, and I am Jan. You are the ideal, and I am the failure. We have both been set up for a classic sibling rivalry with all the ensuing resentment, privilege and angst.

While this can create hostility, it usually just ends up putting us in a defensive mode. We feel like we have to fight to assert our identities as fat people against a mountain of cultural momentum. We have to make space in the world and in our own heads to accommodate the idea that we are okay. Sometimes in the pushback we resort to asserting superiority (e.g. "real women" have curves) or creating a safe space with rules foreign to you. Sometimes we have to process real emotions and decide how to use them constructively. Sometimes we break through the anger and find ourselves respecting other people and their bodies the way we demand others respect us.

So where does all this put our thin allies? After all,

you have a personal, vested effort in making this a world where body diversity is the norm. As a currently thin person you have privilege, but you also have fat friends, family, children, spouses, employers, employees and others affected by prejudice. You may be recovering from or at risk of an eating disorder triggered by our culture's fear of fat. You may gain weight someday and want to be able to still love yourself. You are bombarded every day with messages that your worth to the world and any love you experience is contingent entirely on never allowing your body to change.

But here are some of the ways in which my experience with the same messages is very different. You can go clothes shopping with an expectation that you'll find clothes that express your style in your size at a reasonable price. You won't be mocked by supercilious store employees because you're outside their size range. You will be taken more seriously professionally, and have more opportunity for romantic or sexual involvement. You can join a gym without being pressured to over-exercise to lose weight, and told by staff and other members that your body is unacceptable, or refused service because they're afraid you'll break their machines. You can visit a doctor and have him treat your illness instead of automatically ascribing it to weight and refusing to treat you until you are smaller. You are encouraged (probably from a very young age) to take up space, attract notice, and demand consideration.

You can fight with us to promote body diversity in order to secure rights for everyone, but it does not change your identity or remove your privilege. We fat people recognize that although you choose to support diversity as a thin person, you are already accepted. In fact, you are held up as the ideal. You can't help this any more than I can help being considered the opposite. As Ragen Chastain says, "[T]his is the size I come in." That's what privilege means; you are granted a certain social status based on criteria outside of your reasonable control. You can listen and empathize, but you can't relate. Not on the same level as someone who has actually had the same experience. Your experience has not sensitized you to the nuances and triggers of fat hate. This means that although I love my thin friends, they have the power to hurt me, unwittingly, through even casual comments. Even if they never use that power against me, I can't ignore it.

That's why a thin person can be treated with some ambivalence by fat people in FA. You are in the same outsider status within the FA community as many fat people are outside of the general community. Your thin privilege is no longer effective. This can feel extremely disconcerting or even threatening if you weren't aware of that privilege in the first place. That's why it's so crucial to come into FA with an awareness of the power inequality we all share. You will feel (and be treated) much more like an ally, and less like an outsider.

It is important for you, as a thin person, to acknowledge that trust-building takes time. Some fat people will always be more comfortable around fat friends. Some truly see all people as part of the human family. Some are still struggling with validating their own identity against the ideal you represent. You are welcome at the table, but all parties need patience and understanding in light of the wear and tear on the human soul.

So now that you're at the table, what do you do?

First you must acknowledge that while everyone has some experience with prejudice, every experience is subjective. How a person responds to discrimination depends on personality, resources, and any history of empowerment or lack thereof. Your reaction to appearance pressure cannot be extrapolated to the experiences of a fat person. My experiences as a fat white person cannot be extrapolated to that of a fat Person of Color. Not only do classic identity spectrums such as race, gender, height, age and ability intersect, but many subtle factors can radically change a subjective experience.

Trying to empathize with a fat person by sharing your own discrimination experience is not constructive. It begins a cycle of "more oppressed than thou." You may be trying to relate, but you are actually engaging in one-upmanship and/or attempting to minimize or negate the fat person's experience. You are both excellent witnesses to your own experience and internal life, but they do not compare to anyone else's.

In other words, it's easy to suggest to someone that they stand up to a bully. On the other hand, that person may have decades of intimidation and fear of exposure holding them back. They may have been taught in no uncertain terms that their role in our society is to be invisible and agreeable at all costs. They may have been taught that shame and violence are their only reward for drawing the attention of others. In that context, your "easy" solution becomes a radical act of extraordinary courage.

So be aware of your privilege, especially with close friends who will take what you say and do to heart. If you are going clothes shopping with fat friends, understand that they won't always be able to shop in the same stores, or receive the same service as you do. Respect a friend's discomfort if they don't want to go. You can also put your thin privilege to work here. Clothing stores might not be used to hearing from customers who could be shopping in their stores, but choose not to until they carry quality plus-size lines. Avoid giving money to companies that promote fat-hate in their advertisements and products and let them know why. You are going to be listened to as a customer because you are not as easily dismissed.

But, and this is important, let the fat person's voice be heard. Give us a chance to speak, be visible, and be confident in defending ourselves. Validate our experience. I may be grateful to you for standing up to defend me in a confrontation, but if I'm already doing a good job of it, then take a supporting role. Encourage fat people to speak up through blogs, events and forums instead of speaking for us. Acknowledge that we are the best witness to our experience. This comes down to the concept of self-determinism. We get to define our actions and place in the world. Being dependent on another person to approve us or vouch for us in order to be okay is not okay.

Respect the triggers. When we have become sensitized to insult and prejudice about our weight, it is really easy to send some of us into a spiral of self-loathing or shame. Don't complain about your own weight. Better yet, do your own mental health a favor and eliminate negative body talk altogether. Don't criticize food choices, activity levels, or talk about dieting. Don't ask about my body (i.e. "are you losing weight?") unless I bring it up. If you're unsure as to whether something is offensive, be willing to be corrected and learn from your slips. Allow each person their own identity. It is an absolute insult to tell me I'm not fat when I am obviously, undeniably, unequivocally fat. It's condescending, and denies me the right to come to terms with my body and identity.

You don't have to be fat to be a body-acceptance role model. In addition to respecting triggers and eliminating negative body talk, you can use compliments you're given as educational moments ("Thank you, but I'd look just as good if I wasn't thin/tall/etc."). You can carry it to your doctor's office by demanding they not make assumptions about your health based on your size or even refuse to be weighed unless necessary for dosing medication. Love your body and yourself at the size you come in.

Finally, exercise patience. Remember that many of us are still recovering from very deep emotional wounds. Understand my hurt and anger, and your privilege, and how they color every interaction between us and the world.

Everyone (fat or thin) has a stake and voice in reducing size prejudice in our culture. Even if you are a thin person who takes none of this advice but still believes that I deserve the same human rights as you, then you are part of the solution, and I call you an ally if you wish. We're all in this together and fighting for humanity at every size.

Thin individuals most certainly have a place in fat acceptance, since fat hatred affects everyone in society. A thin person can be an ally and a friend to the movement. Yet the thin person must remember that the fat experience is different.

Men

While the focus of fat acceptance tends to be on women, and women outnumber men in the Fatosphere greatly, fat acceptance is for men, too. To place this in context, eating disorders are increasing in men of all ages, according to the Academy for Eating Disorders. Of those who suffer with anorexia and bulimia, 10 percent are men; additionally, as many as 25 percent of people with a binge eating disorder are men. Some research suggests that gay men are especially vulnerable to eating disorders. One male, William, completed my interview, and explained that fat men require fat acceptance as well:

> I have always been a guy who is more conscious of my weight and how I fit into society. I am quick to take offense when someone who is not a Fat Guy starts [talking] about how accepted Fat Men are in Society compared to Fat Women.

Blogger Nick, writing on the Australian blog *Axis of Fat*, explains that men need a voice in the fat acceptance movement:

> I think fat men of Australia, and the WORLDDDDDD-DD need a voice....I also think there are many fat men out there who, despite seeming very jovial and laughing off the jibes from their "mates", are feeling lost and alone in a world where thin is beautiful and considered normal.

> I've been through depression, the name calling, the school yard taunts, the art of hiding what I eat from people because of the shame. I've lived for years and years doubting that I'm a decent person because I'm fat. I've wondered, "Why me?" and tried all of the diets that I could get my hands on. I've had "caring and thoughtful" family members, friends, work colleagues, internet folk, doctors and people I don't even know suggest that I need to lose a "little" weight.

Fat oppression is not limited to women. In fact, fat men can experience a situation particular to their gender—getting called "big guy." This came up in the original post regarding the Fantasy of Being Thin when Rowan wrote out his fantasy:

> I'm thin, no one will ever use 'big guy' as my default name.
>
> Anytime someone who doesn't know my name wants to address me, from cop to homeless person, that's the name I have. That is all I am. [T]hat descriptor. At this point in my life, I'd almost rather die than have another day when someone calls me that.

Blogger fillyjonk said that her boyfriend received that epithet as well. "I think any mode of address that diminishes the addressee to a single physical attribute," she explained, "whatever it is, really sucks." Rowan also has issues with the term "teddy bear" to explain a man who is "mysteriously attractive and fat at the same time," since it implies that the man is "[a] giant piece of stuffing."

Men and women need fat acceptance equally, and men need a stronger voice in the movement.

Intersectionality

As a Woman of Color, I've felt the pain of knowing that, because of my race, I cannot be beautiful. "Classic beauty" is defined as whiteness. It may be possible to be "unconventionally" attractive, but even that dubious honor tells me my features are abnormal. From this position of pain also comes the opportunity to push back against mainstream standards, and embrace other ideas of beauty. For me, learning to love my fat body is tied up in learning to love my black body. Valuing my thick tightly coiled hair and full lips, has gone hand in hand with loving my rounded belly and big strong thighs.

Julia on *Fatshionista.com*

As the quote above suggests, fat acceptance is for those who have fat bodies that may intersect with other social justice issues—people of color, queer individuals, or those who are other abled, for example. However, these individuals have needs and experiences different than white able-bodied women, needs and experiences that need to be honored and addressed by the movement as a whole.

Attempting to learn from the feminist movement in the 1970s, which ignored the special needs of women of color and lesbian women, many fat acceptance advocates strive to be aware of privilege while balancing the needs of a diverse population—something the white individuals in the movement don't always succeed at. In fact, they have failed spectacularly in past situations.

I realize that this book reflects primarily white, middle class, able-bodied experiences with fat. When I was doing my research, the Fatosphere contained few people of color and disabled individuals speaking out. I'm glad to say that situation is changing, though not to the degree that these populations are being affected by the war on "obesity." To be effective as a movement, fat acceptance must make room for and acknowledge the diverse needs of social justice movements that intersect with fat issues. As sluteverbabe said on her Tumblr:

> [all] oppression is connected but not all oppression is the same, so although we may fight similar struggles we have to respect that some of the oppressions we face are very different from others and give those room to voice our struggle without derailing bullshit

In a 2010 fatcast, Kirby and Kinzel stated that people of color and those who deal with other forms of intersectionality are underrepresented in the Fatosphere. Blogger Julia argues for individuals in fat acceptance to remain aware of other forms of oppression and marginalization:

Fatphobia is just one way in which people are marginalized for having a body that doesn't match societal standards. Many of us are also fighting multiple forms of marginalization and oppression including racism, ableism, transphobia, and homophobia. For me, an important part of Fat Acceptance, and really any movement for social justice, is understanding that ending marginalization for...other groups is an effort that deserves both energy and support. It's also important to accept that some people may prioritize other forms of oppression in their lives, and we shouldn't criticize them for ignoring the "real" problem of fat hatred. We all need to remember that there is no hierarchy of oppression and that none of us can be free when one of us is oppressed.

People of color are some of those most targeted by "anti-obesity" campaigns, as noted on a NOLOSE post about the lack of inclusion of people of color in the 2012 campaign against the Georgia Strong4Life ads:

> [B]oth government programs and the diet industry have been specifically singling out and targeting people of color in recent campaigns. From Michelle Obama's selection of Beyonce Knowles as the face of her national campaign against obese children to the disproportionate number of children of color represented in the state of Georgia's "Strong4Life" campaign, the face of the "obesity epidemic" in public policy has largely become people of color. Similarly, the diet industry has focused several of its most recent national advertising campaigns around African American celebrity icons, including the selection of Janet Jackson as a representative of Nutri System, and Charles Barkley and Jennifer Hudson as spokespeople for Weight Watchers.

In her book *Rock My Soul*, hooks argues that people of color, most especially children, suffer even more because of the white, slender ideal of beauty:

> Since shame about the black body has already been taught by the white Supremacist aesthetics coming from

white media, when fat is added to the picture in a culture where thinness is seen as both a sign of beauty and a sign of well-being, then children suffer.

And yet even when attempting to be conscious of this need for intersectionality, as white-privileged individuals, white fat activists have more to learn. For instance, in 2008 Marilyn Wann led a campaign to send 1,000 fat origami cranes to the Japanese government to protest a move to begin measuring waists of the Japanese people. An anonymous blogger posted a criticism of this project on Kinzel's *Two Whole Cakes* blog:

> The message, to me at least, comes across fairly clearly as we white Americans know better than you, and we'll appropriate your cultural symbols in a (not-at-all racist/ ethnocentric) attempt to help you fix the mess you've gotten yourself into.

Marilyn Wann took this criticism to heart and rethought her activism:

> The 1,000 fat origami cranes project was a wrong, racist, offensive, culturally appropriating bad idea that I should have recognized as a total non-starter. When I started the project, I heard from Charlotte Cooper and I wasn't able to take in the much-deserved criticisms she kindly offered. I realize now that I was horrifyingly prejudicial and hateful in creating the project, working on it, and defending it. I have been distressed about the project for years and have failed to address it publicly...
> I take responsibility for the wrong I did.

> I sincerely regret the harm I've done to individuals and to community.

> I am sorry that people who participated in the project were following my lead. This is not the kind of leadership I want to offer. I will educate myself and make every effort to do better from now on.

Another danger for all fat activists is the tendency to lump people of color together, expecting their experiences to be the same, or at least similar. In response to a *New York Times* editorial by author Alice Randall, writer Jamilah Lemieux wrote the following in *Ebony* magazine:

> We certainly have some specific shared struggles (and sparkles!) as Black people in America, but not all of them look or feel the same. Thus, trying to diagnose or discuss all Black women or men or children as a whole does little more than simply [force] us in a box that is just too small for all of us to fit. Especially the sisters.

It is tempting to talk of the "black experience," "Hispanic experience," or the like as if these populations have no variety within them. In fact, in terms of "Hispanic" populations, in a talk I attended by psychoanalyst Clarissa Pinkola Estés, she explained that "Hispanic" is a term used by a white majority government to lump everyone who speaks Spanish together. These populations tend to have their own preferred terms, such as Latino or Chicana. She suggested asking if you do not know what term they prefer. The temptation to lump groups together must be avoided.

In response to the lack of inclusion regarding people of color in the Strong4Life campaign, NOLOSE POC (People of Color) suggested the following guidelines for working with such intersectionality issues:

- POC in the fat justice movement deserve thoughtful and clear discussions around not just the intention of diversity and inclusion in the work you wish to do, but also the actual impact of the work within communities of color.

- POC in the fat justice movement demand and deserve that white fat activists build authentic collaborations with communities of color and work as allies.

- POC in the fat justice movement demand and deserve allies showing up to the table of our campaigns and work, rather than constantly being told they have made a place for us at theirs.

- POC in the fat justice movement clarify that our allies will practice doing the work of learning about the histories and impacts of colonization and oppression on POC, seek other allies to learn from and with, be open to dialogue, taking feedback, and allowing people's firsthand experiences of racism to be the final and authoritative voice on the subject of impact to communities of color.

- POC in the fat justice movement offer that through the work of authentic inclusivity, singular vision will become shared vision. Coalition will happen. Bridges will be mended and built.

Honestly, I am hesitant to discuss this topic in great detail since I experience white, educated, able-bodied, cisgendered privilege. In fact, one fear that I experience is the fear of "doing it wrong," a fear I know other white activists share to the point that I see white individuals moving away from any form of fat activism out of fear of offending POC and other individuals who deal with intersectionality issues. If white activists make these issues about our fear, we are co-opting such groups' pain. I hesitate to even talk about this fear because, to some degree, making intersectionality about white people's fear is a form of co-opting. At the same time, this fear needs to be addressed.

White activists cannot let that fear keep us from activism. The reality is that fat activists who are white, able-bodied or cisgendered have privilege—privilege that we often cannot even see. What such activists must practice is what Krista Ratcliffe calls "rhetorical listening," "a stance of openness that a person may choose to assume in cross-cultural settings." In other words, such activisits must be open to other points of view as well as open to being called out on privilege.

Privileged activists may make mistakes. When such activisits do make mistakes, they need to accept the criticism and figure out how they can change to make it better next time, as Marilyn Wann showed us in the fat cranes project. In fact, the Tumblr *Racist 101* explains how to address privilege:

> Examples of what white privilege deniers THINK it means to be told to "Check Your Privilege."
>
> Apologize for being white
>
> Believe white is bad or wrong
>
> Be ashamed of being white
>
> Feel guilty for being white
>
> Examples of what people ACTUALLY mean when they say "Check Your Privilege."
>
> You are inserting yourself into a conversation where you shouldn't be. Acknowledge what you are doing, apologize and stop it.
>
> You are making my pain about you. Acknowledge what you are doing, apologize and stop it.
>
> You are belittling my pain. Acknowledge what you are doing, apologize and stop it.
>
> You are making my fears concerns and troubles less important than your annoyance about me talking about my experience. Acknowledge what you are doing, apologize and stop it.

It all comes back to hooks' concept of love. We must seek to understand, appreciate and value each person for their individual qualities and experiences. We must seek to consider everyone's needs and rights. If we started doing this, if we started respecting individuals, we would encounter fewer issues when dealing with a diverse population.

Though I have focused on people of color, the same basic arguments can be made for any other social justice group that intersects with fat activism: LGBT, individuals who are disabled, etc. Intersectionality is an important part of fat acceptance. As noted before, hooks argues that all forms of oppression must be eliminated for oppression to end. Thus, it remains important for individuals in the fat acceptance movement to continue supporting other marginalized groups while being aware of issues surrounding intersectionality.

Non-U.S. Cultures

Fat studies scholar and blogger Charlotte Cooper has taught me that fat acceptance tends to be very American-focused, and that we are not always aware of how fat acceptance works in other countries. She explained the issue in her interview:

> This question makes me think of how Fat Liberation is seen to be located in the US, and that fat activism in "other" countries is marginalised, seen as a secondary afterthought, or measured against an American ideal. In those "other" countries too, Fat is seen as an American import.

Fat acceptance is expanding in many other countries, most notably England and Australia, though I've seen posts by folks around the world.

Fat acceptance is not limited to the United States. Because most of my research was situated in America and was from Americans for the most part, I chose to limit the scope of this book to how fat acceptance works in this country, though I quote from fat activists in other countries. However, American fat activists do need to be conscious and considerate of fat acceptance in other countries and cultures. In these other cultures, fat prejudice and fat activism may not work the same.

Fat individuals in other countries may face different challenges and may have different needs. For instance, fat individuals in England and Australia must negotiate socialized medicine. It is important that fat activists in the United States become aware of and honor the experiences of fat individuals in other cultures.

Everyone Benefits

What these issues show is the need for body autonomy everywhere. Many people in our society feel completely justified in commenting on the bodies of other people, whether it is thinking their opinion should matter to other people, "concern trolling," or simple meanness. All individuals in our culture have the right to exist without having people criticize or comment on their bodies.

So fat acceptance involves everyone: fat and thin, men and women, every sexual identity, every race, every nationality. Beyond just the acceptance of all, there are benefits to the inclusion of variety that a homogenized group will not acquire. For instance, marginality—the location where bi- or multi-cultured individuals often find themselves—provides "the ability to see both cultures more clearly than people who are embedded in any one context," according to Gwyn Kirk and Margo Okazawa-Rey. Another benefit—one I have found to be true and very relevant to my work—is that intersectionality shows the many different flavors of domination and the many similarities. By looking at how many different prejudices work, we can find the keys to domination as a whole.

All humans need body acceptance. "The great majority of women who have benefited in any way from feminist-generated social reforms," hooks argues, "do not want to be seen as advocates of feminism." Similar to hooks' primary argument in her book *Feminism is for Everybody,* fat acceptance is for everyone. Many people do and will benefit from fat acceptance though they may never support it. Because the effort to eliminate "obesity" has affected so many people within the dominant culture in the United States, our culture as a whole will benefit from the cause.

Many fat activists recognize that fat acceptance leads to a more accepting culture overall. Contributors often emphasize that bodies should be loved simply because they are human bodies. Blogger Sweet Machine asks, "Why can't we love the body because we're humans, and humans are embodied?"

CHAPTER 19
Online Environment as a Safe(r) Space

Mostly, my attitude has been shaped by my exposure to the Fat-o-sphere. On a particularly bad day, I [G]oogled something like 'I hate my fat body' and found Shapely Prose. I kept reading and started giving myself and other fat people a break. And seeing us all as human beings.

Interview with Athena

As this quote from Athena suggests, the Fatosphere has been a source of fuel for the fat acceptance movement and a source of love for the fat individual. In this conglomeration of blogs and discussion groups hooks' idea of love is acted out in a number of ways, including a safe space to talk about fat acceptance issues and a source of support.

The Concept of Space

To consider the context of a safe space, we first need to understand that even though the Fatosphere is completely virtual, it is actually a space. Cyberspace is distinct as far as spaces are concerned because it comprises a "different kind of physicality," political science and technology researcher Diana Saco believes, though she argues that there is danger in comparing these spaces in terms of being real and unreal. These spaces are different in that physical space "is present to our bodily senses," while virtual space is a simulation that is not accessible by the body. "The sense that cyberspace is bodiless is the crux of the problem for those skeptics who resist accepting it as a real social space," Saco argues.

Therefore, virtual space is a real space, just a different kind of real space. Barbara Ley, a journalism researcher, found that participants in her study of online mothering and pregnancy support groups made their online community "a place of their own, complete with its own identity, culture, social norms, and group boundaries." Krista Ratcliffe explains how identity can be connected to place by saying, "People are always historically and culturally situated, so too, are their embodied identifications—hence the linkage of identification with place." The Fatosphere as a place, therefore, becomes not only a virtual location but a place for a fat individual to find a sense of connection, community and identity.

Considering that fat liberation is all about the body, the idea of bodiless interaction has some interesting implications. By lurking in the Fatosphere, a newcomer to fat acceptance can explore ideas related to the movement without making themselves known to others, a situation that might be more daunting face to face. This same scenario can apply to individuals who are not fat. Where a person may have to worry about lack of acceptance in a face to face scenario, body size is not an issue online unless the person chooses to make it so. Additionally, it may be that individuals who experience prejudice based on appearance find a safe space in a bodiless environment.

The Concept of Safety

In order to continue looking at the Fatosphere as a safer space, we need to consider the idea of safety. Marianne Kirby and Lesley Kinzel explore the idea of the Fatosphere as a safe space in episode 1.5 of the *Two Whole Cakes* fat cast. A truly safe space does not exist, they argue; the Fatosphere cannot exist without uncomfortable discussions such as the topic of white privilege. Such conversations are essential to the fat acceptance movement and must be addressed when they surface.

On the other hand, they assert that the Fatosphere is a place protected from diet talk and from the dominant message of "fat is bad." Since most of the bloggers control content, they are able to prohibit fat hatred and concern trolling, which allows the Fatosphere to be free from such fat-negative rhetoric.

Communication researchers Malcolm Parks and Kory Floyd argue that online communities do actually provide a safe haven for stigmatized groups.

Community provides the support needed for the individual to resist dominance. To resist can be a challenging and scary experience, yet having a community to support resistance can help tremendously. As hooks says,

> For me this space of radical openness is a margin—a profound edge. Locating oneself there is difficult yet necessary. It is not a "safe" place. One is always at risk. One needs a community of resistance.

Resisting the internalized and external expression of the dominant rhetoric can be a challenge for any individual. However, by being part of a supportive community—the Fatosphere and fat acceptance in the case of fat individuals—the individual can find the power to resist the dominant beliefs.

Public vs. Private

Part of the idea of safety must include the perception of public vs. private spaces. The Fatosphere can appear as a private community, but for the most part it exists in the public domain. In fact, when dealing with uncontrolled public forums, fat acceptance constituents often refer to "sanity watchers' points." The term "sanity watchers" was coined by fillyjonk, parodying Weight Watchers' point system. The use of the term suggests that each individual has a limited number of points each day to deal with fat-phobic comments.

As a result of the control administrators and bloggers assert in the Fatosphere the online community may be a public forum, but it projects a feeling of privacy. We need to be aware of where this concept of public and private meet, hooks emphasizes:

> The public reality and institutional structures of domination make the private space for oppression and exploitation concrete—real. That's why I think it crucial to talk about the points where the public and private meet, to connect the two.

In their book *The Ethics of Internet Research* rhetoricians Heidi McKee and James Porter argue that the concepts of "public" and "private" take on different meanings online, becoming a continuum of grey areas with no clear delineation between the two. These authors assert that the concept of public and private depends upon "the type of venue," which includes the technology being used (blogs, chat rooms, discussion boards, etc.), the way in which the users perceive the space, "the sensitivity of the topics being discussed" and the "vulnerability of the participants."

Most of the technology behind the Fatosphere—blogs, Tumblr, Twitter, etc.—implies a public location. On the other hand, the community tends to cover sensitive topics and, because of prejudice, fat individuals could be considered a vulnerable population. These facts ultimately blur the line between public and private. Therefore, the Fatosphere is somewhere in the grey area of public vs. private.

Love, Support & Online Community

The Fatosphere exemplifies hooks' idea of love in support for the fat individual. Part of this support can be explained by the nature of online communities. Sociologist Sherry Turkle noted that the anonymity of the Web can give the individual a "chance to express often unexplored aspects of the self," an idea seconded by professors Amitai Etzioni and Oren Etzioni. Turkle elaborated by saying that this supports new theories regarding non-pathological and even healthy "multiple selves." We often think of split personalities and schizophrenia when we think of "multiple selves." However, these online multiple selves can be a healthy way for individuals to express their identities. "Online support groups," Ley explains, "are simultaneously social, cultural, technical, and therapeutic spaces."

Through involvement in these communities, fat individuals understand that they have support in facing the many fat negative messages they receive. Kirby claims "to belong to a community of people with similar DANGEROUS RADICAL beliefs so that when I have this experience I know that I am not alone in having this experience;" an ideal that Kinzel agrees with.

Fat individuals find that by being part of a community with a fat-positive culture, they find support. This support creates a dynamic that can provide the fat individuals with self-esteem and confidence to resist external forces perpetuating the dominant fat negative messages, as I explain in the section entitled "The Upward Spiral."

Feeling Left Out

I have found that being involved in the Fatosphere sometimes brings up the old fear of being excluded. Growing up as the fat nerd with no social skills, I often felt left out. Whether it was being picked last, not invited to the party, or being bullied, I had so very many experiences of exclusion as a child that I can be thin-skinned as an adult. In Golda Poretsky's telesummit—a conference via telephone—of fat activists, Marilyn Wann noted that many of us feel this way, that many of us have such experiences, so we can be sensitive to such experiences in the fat acceptance movement.

When I figuratively walked into the Fatosphere, I felt included. Here are my peeps! They understand me. They know what I have been through. Suddenly I had a place where I belonged, which is such a wonderful sensation. No one was looking at my body and saying, "We don't want you here."

The Fatosphere and fat acceptance movement are loving communities. We build each other up. We support each other. We remind each other that we are worthy. And that is the kicker because, as Marianne Williamson says, "[L]ove brings up everything unlike itself." In other words, by loving and being loved, our fears and wounds will surface to be healed. In interacting with this community, I have found my fear of being unwanted can surface.

When these feelings come up, I have a choice. I can run from this fear and let it fester inside me, trying to avoid having it triggered again, which almost always happens. Or I can face it. So far, I have chosen to face it.

What does facing the fear of exclusion look like? I can only speak for myself, but for me it means making a choice. It means choosing to support fat acceptance and the Fatosphere even when I'm feeling outside the circle. It means slogging through the controversies—again—and sticking around anyway. It means recognizing that I will not like everyone in fat acceptance communities and they won't all like me, but understanding we can set aside those differences to work toward a common goal. It means doing my best to make sure others don't feel excluded, yet allow them to heal from their own wounds even if I find watching that painful.

As a child, I was powerless to do anything about feeling excluded. As an adult, I get to make choices.

When I made that choice to be part of this community whether I felt included or not, a sense of freedom overwhelmed me. Now, it will not matter what others do or say—I have made a choice to be included. Now, even if some people have issue with me, I can support the community. Now, I feel included almost always.

CHAPTER 20
The Upward Spiral

From then on it was its own positive feedback loop; the more time I spent hanging out in the FA community, the better I felt about myself, and the more I felt license to be the "me" that I was discovering, and the more I delved into FA and especially HAES.

Interview with car

As this quote from car reveals, resistance communities create an upward spiral of resistance: community acceptance generates self acceptance, which generates resistance toward fat negative messages, which generates more self-acceptance.

When reading hooks' ideas of dominance, resistance appears to be a linear process. First the individual resists the internal belief of inferiority, and then resists the external forces. However, a closer look reveals that resistance follows more of a spiral path than a linear one. Internal resistance provides power for external resistance, making internal resistance easier and providing more strength to resist external forces.

"It is that political movement which most radically addresses the person—the personal," hooks says, "citing the need for transformation of self, of relationships." The political movement assists in transforming the self, which in turn helps the individual to "be better able to act in a revolutionary manner, challenging and resisting domination, transforming the world outside of the self."

In considering this dynamic, hooks linked self-recovery with the need for critical consciousness and resistance. This upward spiral can be understated—it is not obvious at all. But when looking closely into hooks' works as well as the words of participants in fat acceptance, we see that it can be a powerful upward spiral of resistance.

This upward spiral of resistance appeared subtly in focus group participants' discussions of advocacy groups, as well as within the Fatosphere. In the focus group, Rachel noted that she found it easier to accept herself after watching other individuals fight discrimination. Jane added that being involved in an advocacy group helps her "not demonize fat"—not blame fat for her problems, and in turn gives her a language to disagree with others. Vicky identified herself as more than just a fat person after her first NOLOSE conference.

Contributors in the Fatosphere often experience empowerment from reading about fat acceptance. Blog commenter Stacey Stardust explained how she came to speak out about fat acceptance:

> I guess now's as good a time as any to point out that reading about FA and deconstructing the "thin=good, fat=bad" paradigm has really made an incredible difference in my life in terms of being able to talk back to fatphobia, both the outward and the internalized kind.

In response to a Shapeling (the term readers of *Shapely Prose* decided to call themselves) struggling with the idea of giving up the fantasy of being thin, commenter luckyliz suggests finding a new dream and allowing "all the people here give you hope." In a comment on *The Rotund*, Cree says that since joining the

FA community "the world is a completely different place," and these communities have given her a sense of empowerment and agency.

So these online communities of resistance create a reinforcing spiral in their members. As these individuals learn to love themselves, they in turn learn to resist, which gives them more love for themselves. Once more, we see the solution to domination is love.

CHAPTER 21
Love Overall

I really would love for body love, and body acceptance, to be unconditional. I think that, and exactly that, is what we are all feeling the lack of.

mara commenting on *Shapely Prose*

As this quote suggests, hooks' concept of love appears to be a solution to fat prejudice and the problems associated with "obesity" in the dominant culture of the United States. Love can appear as fat or body acceptance, Health at Every Size, or as a safe space in which to be accepted.

However, whether it is private or public, it is political, as previous social justice debates have taught many individuals within the fat acceptance movement. As hooks argues:

[W]e need to concentrate on the politicization of love, not just in the context of talking about victimization in intimate relationships, but in a critical discussion where love can be understood as a powerful force that challenges and resists domination. As we work to be loving, to create a culture that celebrates life, that makes love possible, we move against dehumanization, against domination.

Fear is the source of oppression, hooks asserts, and to move against fear means to choose love: "The choice to love is a choice to connect—to find ourselves in the other." She speaks of this as a "recognition of the Other," which provides a "negotiation that seems to disrupt the possibility of domination."

She calls this a "subject-to-subject" encounter, in contrast to the exercised domination, which looks more like a "subject-to-object" encounter in which the Others are seen as objects rather than individuals within the dominant culture. Krista Ratcliffe asserts that such "conscious identifications…provide grounds for revising identifications troubled by history, uneven power dynamics and ignorance."

As noted in Chapter 14: Hooks vs. Foucault, Foucault saw no solution for domination, but rather suggested that domination will continue to exist. In contrast, hooks argues that the end of domination is possible through love, if both sides are willing.

However, we cannot lose sight that for the fat individual, hooks' concept of love boils down to accepting body diversity—accepting the fat body without need for it to change. As Wann argues, "Weight discrimination will continue to thrive so long as efforts to end it focus on changing people's bodies rather than changing people's minds."

In the case of fat bodies, by examining the dominant rhetoric and resistance to it and by seeking to give voice to the dominated, scholars and fat activists can bring more love into the world.

CONCLUSION
A Truly Just Society

Meanwhile, at this particular moment in time, fat hatred
is not only visible, it is proud of itself.

Ben Spatz on *Cacophony*

Domination/oppression/prejudice——no matter what you call it——
is alive and well in our society in many forms: racism, sexism,
ableism, homophobia, etc. Fat prejudice is one of those forms.
For the most part, this prejudice follows hooks' ideology of
domination. Yet because our society believes that fat is changeable and unhealthy, even many liberals and progressives tend to
believe fat people do not deserve to be protected from dominating forces.

Fat individuals face the same process of internalization that
other oppressed groups face. It follows that their resistance to
such forces should take much of the same shape as other resistance forces. And, in the end, love—connecting to the other—
will prove to be the final solution. However, for the fat individual, this process is complicated by the expectation of change.

We need to transform our entire culture, hooks argues, removing all systems of domination. Our society has established

the same system of domination with fat that we continue to fight with other prejudices. Keeping that in mind, hooks' assertions make a great deal of sense.

Whether it be race, sex, sexual orientation, ableism, another prejudice, or body size, following hooks' arguments we should seek to end all forms of oppression within our society. And rhetoric—persuasion and language—provides the ideal vehicle with which to end these oppressions.

> When we end our silence, when we speak in a liberated voice, our words connect us with anyone, anywhere who lives in silence.
>
> bell hooks

This book has sought to make individuals aware of how oppression works, and to give a voice to those who fight fat oppression, specifically. If we continue to allow any oppression to exist, no matter how compelling the reasons may seem, we are perpetuating domination as a whole.

Until we recognize that fat prejudice cannot be justified, all prejudice will continue to exist. It is time to end fat prejudice and oppression. It is time to end prejudice "for health's sake." It is time to end all prejudice. It is time to end domination in all its forms. In the end, it is time for love to become our driving force.

> Let's be clear that if fat people's "issues with our body size" are actually issues caused by social stigma, then the cure lies in ending social stigma, not ending fat people.
>
> Ragen Chastain

Fat prejudice is not an acceptable prejudice; an acceptable prejudice does not exist. Until we understand this concept, ALL prejudice will continue in some form or another.

NOTES

Chapter 5

"Fat protects a patient post-operatively. 'Overweight' and 'obese' individuals have a decreased risk of death in post-surgical ICU." Hutagalung et al. found this to be true in "The obesity paradox in surgical intensive care unit patients," published in the *Journal of Intensive Care Medicine.*

"Obese patients with type 2 diabetes have lower mortality rates, meaning they live longer." This information can be found in Doehner et al.'s "Inverse relation of body weight and weight change with mortality and morbidity in patients with type 2 diabetes and cardiovascular co-morbidity: An analysis of the PROactive study population," published in the *International Journal of Cardiology.*

"Higher mortality is associated with weight loss in type 2 diabetic patients, yet weight gain did not change mortality rates." This information can also be found in Doehner et al.'s "Inverse relation of body weight and weight change with mortality and morbidity in patients with type 2 diabetes and cardiovascular co-morbidity: An analysis of the PROactive study population" published in the *International Journal of Cardiology.*

"'Obese' individuals with type 2 diabetes have less incidences of amputation. Additionally, they experience better post-operative outcomes after amputation." Sohn et al. discussed this in "Obesity paradox in amputation risk among nonelderly diabetic men," published in the journal *Obesity.*

"Being 'overweight' or 'obese' lowers the mortality rate for those with cardiovascular disease." Romero-Corral et al.'s "Association of bodyweight with total mortality and with cardiovascular events in coronary artery disease: a systematic review of cohort studies," published in *Lancet.*

"'Obesity' protects against respiratory failure in post-operative patients." Donohoe et al. found this to be true in "Perioperative evaluation of the obese patient," published in the *Journal of Clinical Anesthesia.*

"'Obese' dialysis patients have better survival outcomes." This was discussed in Kalantar-Zadeh et al.'s "Survival advantages of obesity in dialysis patients," published in the *American Journal of Clinical Nutrition.*

"COPD patients with a higher BMI live longer." More on COPD patients can be found in Memtsoudis et al.'s "Mortality of patients with respiratory insufficiency and adult respiratory distress syndrome after surgery: The obesity paradox," published in the *Journal of Intensive Care Medicine.*

"A number of studies reveal that fat individuals have better outcomes after a stroke." Scherbakov et al.'s "Body weight after stroke: Lessons from the obesity paradox," published in the journal *Stroke,* Ovbiagele et al.'s "Obesity and recurrent vascular risk after a recent ischemic stroke," published in the journal *Stroke,* and Katsnelson et al.'s "Obesity paradox and stroke: Noticing the (fat) man behind the curtain," also published in *Stroke.*

"Weight gain has been associated with lower mortality rates while weight loss has been associated with higher mortality rates." Myers et al. found this to be true in "The obesity paradox and weight loss," published in the *American Journal of Medicine.*

"This result was found in three independent studies that

took place in the United States, in Canada, and in Japan." Studies that reached the conclusion that overweight individuals live the longest include Flegal, K. M., Graubard, B. I., Williamson, D. F., & Gail, M. H. (2005). Excess deaths associated with underweight, overweight, and obesity. *Journal of the American Medical Association,* 293(15), 1861-1867; "BMI and all-cause mortality among Japanese older adults: findings from the Japan collaborative cohort study" by Tamakoshi et al. and "Results from a national longitudinal study of Canadian adults" by Orpana et al., both published in the journal *Obesity.*

"We know that dieting causes horrible effects to the body, including gall stones and increases in cortisol level." Shiffman, Sugerman, Kellum, Brewer, & Moore found that dieting caused gall stones in the article "Gallstone formation after rapid weight loss: A prospective study in patients undergoing gastric bypass surgery for treatment of morbid obesity," published in the *American Journal of Gastroenterology.*

"Also, 40 percent of doctors have been found to have to weight prejudice." Kalet et al. found weight prejudice among physicians in the study "Physicians' attitudes about obesity and their associations with competency and specialty: A cross-sectional study," published in *BMC Health Services Research.*

Chapter 6

"Preschool aged children already have anti-fat bias, while those with a caregiver who have anti-fat attitudes have higher levels of anti-fat bias." Rich et al. looked at Hispanic children's perception of fat in "Predictors of body size stigmatization in Hispanic preschool children," published in the journal *Obesity.*

"As many as 25 percent of adolescents report weight-based teasing throughout their adolescent years by their peers, and 48 percent report teasing by both peers and family, with obese adolescents report significantly higher incidence of teasing." Haines, Neumark-Sztainer, Hannan, van den Berg, & Eisenberg published their article "Longitudinal and secular trends in weight-related teasing during adolescence" in the journal *Obesity* in 2008.

Chapter 7

"Access to healthy foods is often limited in poverty stricken areas..." Information on access to healthy foods can be found in L.M. Powella, S. Slaterb, D. Mirtchevaa, Y. Baoa, & F.J. Chaloupka's 2007 article "Food store availability and neighborhood characteristics in the United States," published in *Preventive Medicine*.

"Fat women are also more likely to experience mistreatment at the hands of strangers than are fat men." This information can be found in the article "Mistreatment due to weight: prevalence and sources of perceived mistreatment in women and men" by N.H. Falkner, S.A. French, R.W. Jeffery, D. Neumark-Sztainer, N.E. Sherwood, & N. Morton, published in *Obesity Research* in 1999.

"Not only are eating disorders increasing at an alarming rate in teenage girls..." Bonnie Spear discussed such eating disorder issues in her 2006 article "Does dieting increase the risk for obesity and eating disorders?" published in the *Journal of the American Dietetic Association*.

"...they are increasing in women and men of all ages." The Academy for Eating Disorders says that eating disorders are increasing in everyone (http://www.aedweb.org/eating_disorders/prevalence.cfm).

"...up to 30 percent of girls are estimated to have disordered eating habits." This information also comes from Spear's article, noted above.

"One of the primary precursors to the prevalence of eating disorders is the incidence of weight loss dieting." This was also found in Spear's article.

"Body dissatisfaction, not weight itself, increases suicide risks in girls." R. Nauert notes this fact in "Perceptions can drive teen suicide behaviors," published in 2009 on PsychCentral. com.

Chapter 8

"Evidence that fat individuals are seen as inferior can be found everywhere from school classrooms to doctor's offices, in the media, and in daily life." Information on inferiority found in the classroom can be found in J. Weinstock & M. Krehbiel's article in *The Fat Studies Reader:* "Fat Youth as Common Targets for Bullying." Jay et al. found that physicians tended to be biased toward fat individuals in their 2009 article "Physicians' attitudes about obesity and their associations with competency and specialty: A cross-sectional study," published in *BMC Health Services Research.* Information on fat individuals seen as inferior in the media can be found in D. Giovanelli & S. Ostertag's "Controlling the body: Media representations, body size, and self-discipline," published in *The Fat Studies Reader.* Information on fat people seen as inferior in daily life can be found in "Bias, Discrimination, and Obesity," written by Rebecca Puhl &Kelly Brownell and published in *Obesity Research.* Such information can also be found in Puhl and Brownell's "Confronting and coping with weight stigma: An investigation of overweight and obese individuals," published in the journal *Obesity.*

"Since parents, especially mothers, are often blamed for their children being fat..." Boero argued that mothers are often blamed for fat in "Fat Kids, Working Moms, and the 'Epidemic of Obesity': Race, Class and Mother Blame" in *The Fat Studies Reader.*

Chapter 10

"Even fat individuals have a strong anti-fat bias, starting at as young as three years old." Schwartz, Vartanian, Nosek, & Brownell found that fat individuals have a strong anti-fat bias in their 2006 article "The influence of one's own body weight on implicit and explicit anti-fat bias," published in the journal *Obesity*. Cramer & Steinwert found anti-fat bias in children documented in their article "Thin is good, fat is bad: How early does it begin?" published in the *Journal of Applied Developmental Psychology*.

"This self hate is so prevalent that children as young as five are starting to have body image issues." Davison, Schmalz, Young, & Birch reported body image issues in children in their 2008 article "Overweight girls who internalize fat stereotypes report low psychosocial well-being," published in the journal *Obesity*.

Chapter 13

"However, fat individuals often find this to be very difficult, since they are often perceived as lazy and slovenly." Schwartz, Chambliss, Brownell, Blair, & Billington found this perception of fat individuals in their article "Weight bias among health professionals specializing in obesity," published in the journal *Obesity Research*.

"Lesley explains that she took the name from the medical term 'morbidly obese,' which the medical establishment defines as 'being in excess of 100 pounds or 100 percent over maximum recommended weight.'" Fikkan & Rothblum reported this definition of 'morbid obesity' in the chapter entitled "Weight bias in employment" in the book *Weight Bias: Nature, Consequences, and Remedies*.

Chapter 15

"When considering knowledge creation in online environments, the first thing to understand is that such 'knowledge is always situated,' and since online experiences 'disrupt the sense of bounded space...'" B. Smith argued that knowledge is situated in "Researching hybrid literacies: Methodological explorations of ethnography and the practices of the cybertariat" in McKee & DeVoss's *Digital Writ-*

ing Research: Technologies, Methodologies and Ethical Issues.

Chapter 16

"When an online discussion of research showing that fat individuals can be healthy..." Stefan, Kantartzis, Machann, Schick, Thamer, Rittig, and others found that many fat individuals are healthy in "Identification and characterization of metabolically benign obesity in humans," published in *Archives of Internal Medicine.*

Chapter 18

"Of those who suffer with anorexia and bulimia, 10 percent are men and as many as 25 percent of those with binge eating disorder are men." Research on men with eating disorders comes from Weltzin, Weisensel, Franczyk, Burnett, Klitz, & Bean's article "Eating disorders in men: Update," published in the *Journal of Men's Health & Gender.*

"Some research suggests that gay men are especially vulnerable to eating disorders." Russell & Keel found that gay men may be vulnerable to eating disorders in "Homosexuality as a specific risk factor for eating disorders in men," published in the *International Journal of Eating Disorders.*

"...learning from the feminist movement in the 1970s, which ignored the special needs of women of color and lesbian women..." The topic is discussed in the textbook *Women's Lives: Multicultural Perspectives* by Kirk & Okazawa-Rey.

Fat Studies Books & Articles

Bacon, Linda. (2010). *Health At Every Size: The Surprising Truth About Your Weight.* Dallas, Tx: Benbella Books, Inc.

Bacon, L., Stern, J. S., Loan, M. D. V., & Keim, N. L. (2005). Size acceptance and intuitive eating improve health for obese, female chronic dieters. *Journal of the American Dietetic Association,* 105, 929-936.

Campos, P. F. (2004). *The Diet Myth: Why America's Obsession with Weight Is Hazardous to Your Health.* New York, NY: Penguin Group (USA), Inc.

Campos, P. F., Saguy, A., Ernsberger, P., Oliver, J. E., & Gaesser, G. A. (2006). The epidemiology of overweight and obesity: public health crisis or moral panic? *International Journal of Epidemiology,* 35(1), 55-60.

Fraser, L. (1997). *Losing It: America's Obsession with Weight and the Industry that Feeds on It.* New York, NY: Dutton Adult.

Gaesser, G. A. (1999). Thinness and weight loss: Beneficial or detrimental to longevity. *Medicine and Science in Sports and Exercise,* 31(8), 118-1128.

Gaesser, G. A. (2002). *Big Fat Lies: The Truth About Your Weight and Your Health.* Carlsbad, CA: Gurze Books.

Gaesser, G. A. (2003). Is it necessary to be thin to be healthy? *Harvard Health Policy Review,* 4(2), 40-47.

Gard, M. (2005). *The Obesity Epidemic: Science, Morality and Ideology.* New York, NY: Routledge.

Harding, K., and Kirby, M. (2009). *Lessons from the Fat-o-sphere: Quit Dieting and Declare a Truce With Your Body.* New York, New York: Penguin Group (USA), Inc.

Hirschmann, J. R., and Munter, C. H. (1995). *When Women Stop Hating Their Bodies.* New York: Fawcett Books.

Kolata, G. (2007). *Rethinking Thin: The New Science of Weight Loss—and the Myths and Realities of Dieting.* New York: Farrar, Straus, and Giroux.

Oliver, J. E. (2006a). *Fat Politics: The Real Story Behind America's Obesity Epidemic.* USA: Oxford University Press.

Oliver, J. E. (2006b). The politics of pathology: How obesity became an epidemic disease. *Perspectives in Biology and Medicine,* 49(4), 611-627.

Rothblum, E., & Solovay, S.(Eds.) (2009). *The Fat Studies Reader.* New York and London: New York University Press.

Saguy, A., & Ward, A. (2010). Coming out as fat: Rethinking stigma. *Social Psychology Quarterly,* March 2011, 74(1). 53-75.

Saguy, A. C., & Almeling, R. (2008). Fat in the fire? Science, the news media, and the "obesity epidemic." *Sociological Forum,* 23(1), 53-83.

Solovay, S. (2000). *Tipping the Scales of Justice: Fighting Weight-Based Discrimination.* New York: Prometheus Books.

Wann, M. (1999). *Fat!So?: Because You Don't Have to Apologize for Your Size!* Berkeley, CA: Ten Speed Press.

Fat Positive Internet Resources

Big Fat Blog:
www.bigfatblog.com/

Fat Body Politics Tumblr:
http://fatbodypolitics.tumblr.com/

Fat Positive/HAES Marketing Facebook group:
http://www.facebook.com/groups/207243959295384/

Fat Studies Facebook group:
http://www.facebook.com/groups/5565108314/

Health At Every Size blog:
http://healthateverysizeblog.org/

Health At Every Size community:
http://www.haescommunity.org

Hey, fat chick! Tumblr:
http://heyfatchick.tumblr.com/

Kath Read's *Fat Heffalump* blog:
http://fatheffalump.wordpress.com/

Lara Frater's *Fat Chicks Rule!* blog:
http://fatchicksrule.blogs.com/fat_chicks_rule/

Linda Bacon's website:
http://www.lindabacon.org/

Living ~400 lbs **blog:**
http://living400lbs.wordpress.com/

Marianne Kirby's *The Rotund* **blog:**
http://therotund.com

Ragen Chastain's *Dances with Fat* **blog:**
http://danceswithfat.wordpress.com/

The Well Rounded Mama **blog:**
http://wellroundedmama.blogspot.com/

For updated links, see
http://www.loniemcmichael.com/fatlinks

About the Author

Lonie McMichael has wanted to be a writer since age 3. For many years she practiced her trade as a technical writer in the high tech industry. After going to graduate school, Lonie found her calling in fat studies, exploring the fat individual's experience. Graduating with a Ph.D. in technical communication and rhetoric, she wrote her dissertation on the medical rhetoric surrounding the "obesity epidemic" and how such rhetoric legitimizes fat prejudice—topics which have become two separate books, *Talking Fat* and *Acceptable Prejudice?* (the former published by Pearlsong Press in 2012).

She is currently teaching professional and technical writing at the University of Colorado at Colorado Springs and working on her third book about things fat. Visit her on the web at www.loniemcmichael.com.

A BOOK GROUP STUDY GUIDE TO *ACCEPTABLE PREJUDICE?*
can be downloaded at
www.pearlsong.com/acceptableprejudice.htm.

About Pearlsong Press

Pearlsong Press is an independent publishing company dedicated to providing books and resources that entertain while expanding perspectives on the self and the world. The company was founded by Peggy Elam, Ph.D., a psychologist and journalist, in 2003.

We encourage you to enjoy other Pearlsong Press books, which you can purchase at www.pearlsong.com or your favorite bookstore. Keep up with us through our blog at www.pearlsongpress.com.

FICTION:

Fatropolis—a paranormal adventure by Tracey L. Thompson
The Falstaff Vampire Files—paranormal adventure by Lynne Murray
Larger Than Death, Large Target, At Large & A Ton of Trouble—
Josephine Fuller mysteries by Lynne Murray
The Season of Lost Children—a novel by Karen Blomain
Fallen Embers & *Blowing Embers*—Books 1 & 2 of The Embers
Series, paranormal romance by Lauri J Owen
The Fat Lady Sings—a young adult novel by Charlie Lovett
Syd Arthur—a novel by Ellen Frankel
Bride of the Living Dead—romantic comedy by Lynne Murray
Measure By Measure—a romantic romp with the fabulously fat
by Rebecca Fox & William Sherman
FatLand—a visionary novel by Frannie Zellman
The Program—a suspense novel by Charlie Lovett
The Singing of Swans—a novel about the Divine Feminine
by Mary Saracino

ROMANCE NOVELS & SHORT STORIES FEATURING BIG BEAUTIFUL HEROINES:

by Pat Ballard, the Queen of Rubenesque Romances:
Dangerous Love | *The Best Man* | *Abigail's Revenge*

Dangerous Curves Ahead: Short Stories | *Wanted: One Groom*
Nobody's Perfect | *His Brother's Child* | *A Worthy Heir*
by Rebecca Brock—*The Giving Season*
& by Judy Bagshaw—*Kiss Me, Nate!* & *At Long Last, Love*

Nonfiction:

Hiking the Pack Line: Moving from Grief to a Joyful Life—
by Bonnie Shapbell
A Life Interrupted: Living with Brain Injury—
poetry by Louise Mathewson
ExtraOrdinary: An End of Life Story Without End—
memoir by Michele Tamaren & Michael Wittner
Love is the Thread: A Knitting Friendship by Leslie Moïse, Ph.D.
Fat Poets Speak: Voices of the Fat Poets' Society—Frannie Zellman, Ed.
Ten Steps to Loving Your Body (No Matter What Size You Are)
by Pat Ballard
Beyond Measure: A Memoir About Short Stature & Inner Growth
by Ellen Frankel
*Taking Up Space: How Eating Well & Exercising Regularly Changed
My Life* by Pattie Thomas, Ph.D. with Carl Wilkerson, M.B.A.
(foreword by Paul Campos, author of *The Obesity Myth*)
*Off Kilter: A Woman's Journey to Peace with Scoliosis, Her Mother
& Her Polish Heritage*—a memoir by Linda C. Wisniewski
Unconventional Means: The Dream Down Under—
a spiritual travelogue by Anne Richardson Williams
Splendid Seniors: Great Lives, Great Deeds—
inspirational biographies by Jack Adler

Healing the World One Book at a Time